Manual for the Videofluorographic Study of Swallowing

Manual for the Videofluorographic Study of Swallowing

SECOND EDITION

Jeri A. Logemann

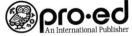
pro·ed
An International Publisher

8700 Shoal Creek Boulevard
Austin, Texas 78757-6897
800/897-3202   Fax 800/397-7633
www.proedinc.com

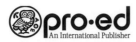

© 1986, 1993 by PRO-ED, Inc.
8700 Shoal Creek Boulevard
Austin, Texas 78757-6897
800/897-3202   Fax 800/397-7633
www.proedinc.com

Library of Congress Cataloging-in-Publication Data

Logemann, Jeri A., 1942–
    Manual for the videofluorographic study of swallowing / Jeri A.
Logemann.
      p.   cm.
    Rev. ed. of: 1986.
    Includes bibliographical references and index.
    ISBN 0-89079-584-3
    1. Deglutition disorders—Diagnosis.   2. Videofluoroscopy.
I. Title.
RC815.2.L635   1993
616.3'1—dc20

                               92-41623
                                 CIP

This book is designed in 11 on 13 Bodoni with Helvetica

Printed in the United States of America

      7   8   9   10   07 06

Table of Contents

Preface

Since the first edition of this manual was published in 1986, our knowledge of normal swallowing physiology has advanced, resulting in changes in the procedure of the modified barium swallow as well as changes in interpretation of some of its aspects.

This edition of the manual is designed to present the latest rationale and procedures for the modified barium swallow, to describe the variations on the typical modified barium swallow that make it a more valuable evaluation technique, and to define and describe oropharyngeal swallowing disorders. The videofluorographic worksheet at the back of the manual is intended to complement this discussion and facilitate interpretation of the modified barium swallow. This edition provides much expanded information on normal swallowing physiology (Chapter 2) and its variations in infants and older adults and on ways to measure normal and abnormal swallowing physiology (Chapter 6) as part of diagnosis, as well as on the measurement of treatment efficacy. The description of the modified barium swallow procedure (Chapter 3) has been broadened to incorporate testing of liquid bolus volume changes if tolerated by the patient. This inclusion reflects the recognition of the extent to which bolus volume affects normal swallowing and can affect the dysphagic patient (for better or worse). The importance of bedside clinical assessment of the patient's swallowing before the modified barium swallow is conducted is discussed in Chapter 1.

Suggestions for management and therapy procedures that can be introduced into the radiographic study to improve swallowing safety or efficiency in patients with various swallowing disorders are detailed in Chapter 4, as are other variations on the "standard" modified barium swallow procedure. These variations have expanded dramatically since the first edition of this manual, as have the patient populations for whom the procedure is needed. Chapter 4 also describes the particular preparations and adaptations needed to produce a valid and successful radiographic study in these special populations. For further descriptions of treatment suggestions for various swallowing disorders, the reader is referred to the text *Evaluation and Treatment of Swallowing Disorders* (Logemann, 1983) and the articles referenced therein and at the back of this manual.

After describing the modified barium swallow procedure and its variations, each oropharyngeal swallowing disorder is described according to its radiographic symptoms (Chapter 5). Many are illustrated with still radiographic films, videoprints, and tracings from these films. Clinical decision making used during the radiographic study to introduce management strategies is illustrated for various swallowing disorders in Chapter 7. Recommendations that can be made from the modified barium swallow are outlined in Chapter 8. Examples of reports from the modified barium swallow are included in Chapter 9 for inpatients and outpatients with a variety of medical diagnoses. Appendix A is designed to serve as a resource for clinicians looking to purchase pieces of equipment or supplies to use in performing the modified barium swallow. Prices are not provided because they change frequently, but names and addresses of manufacturers are included. The Videofluorographic Worksheet (Appendix B) at the end of this manual summarizes these swallowing disorders and symptoms and is designed to structure observations of anatomy and physiology of the upper aerodigestive tract made during the modified barium swallow study.

Overall, this manual is designed as a pragmatic resource for clinicians evaluating oropharyngeal dysphagic patients by using videofluoroscopy. It should be helpful in designing and implementing the radiographic study with a wide range of patients including those who can be difficult to examine, such as children, head-injured patients, and those with movement disorders.

Acknowledgments

I would like to thank a number of individuals who have assisted in the production of this book. Mary Rooney tirelessly typed numerous revisions of the manuscript. Lee Mendoza checked innumerable details in the production. Cathy Lazarus, Sharon Veis, Liz Bisch, and Terry Shanahan contributed to the patient management issues presented herein. Barbara Pauloski, Joan Cheng, Masako Fujiu, Pat Gibbons, and Peter Kahrilas assisted me in developing the research foundation for the clinical procedures described. Particular thanks go to Hilda Fisher, Barbara Pauloski, and Cathy Lazarus for time in reading, challenging, and collaborating on the contents of this manuscript.

Jeri A. Logemann

Assessment of Need and Readiness for the Modified Barium Swallow

Role of the Bedside Clinical Assessment of Swallowing

As dysphagia is recognized earlier after admission in the acutely ill hospitalized patient or the nursing home population, the question of when to bring the patient to radiology for a modified barium swallow (MBS) arises. A bedside swallowing assessment should precede a radiographic evaluation. In this way, patients who are inappropriate for the radiographic study can be identified and managed at the bedside until their medical status, behavior, or cognitive level enables them to have a radiographic study. In addition to determining the patient's readiness and/or need for a radiographic study, a bedside clinical assessment of swallowing completed before the radiographic assessment can provide the clinician with important information regarding how to best prepare for and manage the patient during the radiographic assessment. Specifically, the bedside examination will provide information regarding the locus of the patient's dysphagia, that is, whether it is oral or pharyngeal; the patient's readiness for a radiographic study; the patient's ability to accept food into the mouth; the oral reaction to placement of various tastes, temperatures, and textures in the oral cavity; the presence of any swallowing apraxia or any abnormal oral reflexes such as the tonic bite; and any particular postural and behavioral needs of the patient that must be addressed during the radiographic study.

By doing a bedside or clinical swallowing assessment before the radiographic examination, the clinician may be able to circumvent some difficulties in radiology and succeed in obtaining better data regarding the patient's swallowing function.

The bedside examination for an in- or outpatient should contain a complete review of the patient's medical history including:

1. Current and past medical problems, focusing on those that may cause dysphagia

2. Current and recently taken medications

3. History of the swallowing disorder, including time and nature of its onset, symptoms such as coughing or food "catching" in the pharynx, difficult and easy foods, and the patient's general perception and awareness of the problem

4. Presence, type, and duration of placement of any airway device (tracheostomy, mechanical ventilation, intubation)

5. Presence, type, and duration of placement and adequacy of oral and non-oral nutrition

6. Observation of secretion levels and the patient's awareness and management of these secretions, including drooling, gurgly voice, and chest secretions

7. Patient's general level of awareness, cognition, and receptive and expressive language

8. Oral anatomy and location of any pooled secretions

9. Assessment of motor control of lips, tongue, palate, pharynx, and larynx

10. Evaluation of the gag and palatal reflexes

11. Examination of oral sensation using light touch

12. Trial feeding of selected small boluses if deemed safe and appropriate

Patients with suspected pharyngeal dysphagia are most appropriate for the X-ray study. Bedside symptoms suggestive of a pharyngeal dysphagia include: reduced pharyngeal or laryngeal function on bedside assessment; repeated pneumonia; weight loss of unknown etiology; gurgly voice quality, especially after eating; suspected delay in triggering the pharyngeal swallow or reduced laryngeal elevation observed on bedside assessment; obvious difficulty eating or slow eating in the presence of functional tongue motion; and coughing during or after swallowing (Horner, Massey, Riski, Lathrop, & Chase, 1988; Linden & Siebens, 1983; Logemann, 1983). Patients with certain medical diagnoses are at high risk for pharyngeal dysphagia and should have an MBS if symptoms of dysphagia are noted. These include: patients with brain-stem stroke, head injury, or spinal cord injury with anterior cervical fusion; tracheotomized patients; mechanically ventilated patients; partial laryngectomees (hemilaryngectomees and supraglottic laryngectomees); patients with surgical resection of part of the posterior-lateral oral cavity including tonsil or tongue base, skull base resection, and resection for acoustic neuroma; and patients with motor neuron disease, Parkinson's disease, multiple sclerosis, and myasthenia gravis (Blonsky, Logemann, Boshes, & Fisher, 1978; Donner & Silbiger, 1966; Lazarus & Logemann, 1987; Logemann, 1985, 1986, 1989a, 1989b; McConnel, Mendelsohn, & Logemann, 1986, 1987; Robbins, 1987; Robbins, Logemann, & Kirshner, 1986; Veis & Logemann, 1985).

If the bedside assessment reveals only oral problems, a radiographic evaluation is probably not needed. Therapy can be planned from the results of the bedside assessment. If behavioral problems or dementia are the primary causes of dysphagia, a radiographic study is usually not needed. And if the patient has no recovery potential and cannot follow directions or comply with compensatory strategies, a radiographic study is not appropriate.

Patient's Readiness for Radiographic Study

In order to complete a radiographic study successfully, a patient should be alert, awake, and able to accept food into the mouth in a reasonably normal length of time. If patients are extremely sleepy or inconsistent in their level of alertness, they frequently exhibit a delayed triggering of the pharyngeal swallow (swallowing reflex). They are often incapable of oral intake sufficient for nutrition or hydration, even if their swallow is functional, because of their inconsistent alertness, inability to focus on the task, or fatigue. Such patients should wait for a radiographic study until they are consistently alert.

There may be exceptions to this general criterion if the patient is suspected of aspirating his or her own secretions or if there are other medical reasons why it is important to understand the patient's oropharyngeal swallowing function. Medically unstable patients should be accompanied to Radiology by medical support (a nurse, physician, or respiratory therapist) and observed throughout the procedure.

Ability to Accept Food into the Mouth

In order to complete the radiographic study, the patient should not be severely orally defensive and should be able to open his or her mouth in a reasonable length of time. Some infants and young children and cognitively impaired adults pull away from a spoon or food approaching their mouth because of lack of visual recognition of the object, previous severe problems with swallowing, or poor management, such as force-feeding or other negative experiences with food. These individuals require desensitization to eliminate their oral defensiveness prior to conducting the radiographic study. It is important for clinicians not to force the patient to accept food into the mouth. The radiographic study and swallowing therapy should not be associated with negative oral reactions, since the patient may need to be reevaluated and this negative association will make reevaluation more difficult. In some cases, desensitization therapy may be needed over a period of a week or two before the radiographic study can be accomplished. For many patients, a short 2 to 3 minutes of desensitization using an empty spoon, as described in the section on Special Populations in Chapter 4, will frequently eliminate the defensiveness.

Ability to Open the Mouth Voluntarily

For some patients with head injury or severe neurologic impairment, voluntary mouth opening is difficult and slow, taking 3 to 5 minutes (Logemann, 1986). Many of these patients are not ready for radiographic assessment of their swallow because of the severity of their neurologic damage and their slow recovery. These patients may benefit most from bedside assessment with oromotor stimulation, including work on control of mouth opening, rather than from an immediate radiographic study. The radiographic study can be scheduled when the patient is able to open his or her mouth more easily.

In some of these patients, however, there is a question of aspiration of secretions, and a radiographic assessment is requested. In this situation, the patient will usually need oral massage to achieve mouth opening. In general, a combination of rotary massage of the cheek (masseter muscle) on one side, with firm downward pressure on the chin, and verbal reinforcement over several minutes will enable the patient to achieve mouth opening in the fluoroscopic suite. As the patient's mouth opens, the clinician should determine whether a bite reflex is present. This can be done by using a 4-by-4-in. gauze roll to touch the teeth and alveolar ridge. Using the gauze prevents the patient from breaking a tooth or biting off a piece of the gauze if a bite reflex is present. In patients with a bite reflex, a spoon that does not break or splinter easily (usually a Mothercare spoon) should be used to place food in the patient's mouth. If possible, the clinician should avoid touching the spoon against the patient's teeth or alveolar ridge. In some cases, this is difficult because the patient can only achieve a limited mouth opening. Usually, however, with massage and verbal reinforcement to provide the patient with feedback regarding his or her success in achieving mouth opening, and time allocated to achieve mouth opening, the radiographic study can be performed on at least enough swallows to determine whether or not aspiration occurs and why. In this way, the physiology of the oropharyngeal swallow and etiology of aspiration can be identified, which is critical in planning treatment. The radiographic study is designed not only to identify the symptoms of swallow disorders such as aspiration, but to identify their physiologic or anatomic etiology so that adequate treatment can be provided.

Identification of Optimal Oral Stimuli and Bolus Types

Some cognitively impaired patients will produce more oral activity in response to particular combinations of taste, texture, and temperature. At the bedside, the clinician can use 4-by-4-inch pieces of cloth including gauze, burlap, and satin, rolled around a flexible plastic straw, to present various textures in the mouth. One end of these materials can be dipped into liquid of various temperatures (such as cold or room temperature) and flavors (such as sour, sweet, bitter, or salty) to present a variety of stimuli in the patient's oral cavity. Using a variety of combinations of taste, temperature, and texture, the clinician can identify the particular combination of stimuli that elicits the most oral movements that are characteristic of a normal oropharyngeal swallow. These stimuli (mixed with barium) can then be introduced in X Ray as the bolus. In this way, during the radiographic study, the clinician can assess the patient's reaction to the stimuli identified at the bedside as optimal, in addition to presenting as many of the calibrated boluses included in the standard protocol as possible.

Identification of and Compensation for Swallowing Apraxia

Patients with swallowing apraxia will usually perform best at the bedside when no verbal directions are given regarding eating or swallowing (Tuch & Nielsen, 1941). When a food tray is presented to these patients without verbal instruction, they often pick up the fork or spoon and begin feeding themselves normally with apparently normal swallowing. In contrast, when these patients are brought to X Ray, they often have severe difficulty initiating the oral stage of swallowing to the point of no oral movement because verbal commands are given regarding when to swallow. The more consciously these patients are focused on the swallowing act, the more difficulty they have producing a swallow. If the clinician is aware that a patient is apraxic before the radiographic exam, food may be given to that patient in Radiology without any verbal command, or patients may be given a spoon and a dish of food to feed themselves. If a patient shows only apraxia and no other swallowing disorder, particularly in the pharynx, a radiographic study is not needed.

Identification of and Compensation for Abnormal Oral Reflexes

Some neurologically impaired patients exhibit abnormal oral reflexes such as a hyperactive gag, tongue thrusting, or tonic bite (Logemann, 1989b). These reflexes are usually counterproductive to the acceptance of food in the mouth and the production of a normal swallow. At the bedside, these abnormal reflexes can be identified, and techniques to avoid eliciting them or to desensitize them can be introduced prior to bringing the patient for the radiographic study. Identification of the location in the mouth where these reflexes are triggered and the nature of the stimuli that trigger them is important, so that they can be avoided during the X-ray protocol. Use of a heavy plastic spoon, such as a Mothercare spoon, is recommended for use in the radiographic study with patients who have a bite reflex.

Identification of Particular Postural or Behavioral Needs

Each patient's typical posture during eating should be observed and noted so that it . can be re-created as closely as possible during the radiographic study. If a patient has a postural restriction, such as a spinal cord injury, and can be elevated only to 30° or 60°, these restrictions should be noted and followed in X Ray. Some patients require special wheelchairs or other seating devices that must be accommodated during the radiographic study.

Some patients exhibit behavioral problems requiring accommodation in the radiographic study. For example, some head-injured patients and children react negatively to noises of any kind. Before an MBS can be completed successfully with these patients, they may need to observe a radiographic study done with another patient, so that they can become familiar with the sounds of the equipment as well as the staff involved.

Patient and Family Counseling Regarding Expectations of the Radiographic Study

Many dysphagic patients and their families have unrealistic expectations of the radiographic study. The patient and/or family may assume that the patient will be able to eat after the X-ray study, while the clinician may be performing the radiographic study only to identify the patient's swallowing disorder and define a treatment plan, .intending to keep the patient nonoral. It is important that the clinician counsel the patient and family regarding the purpose and goals of the radiographic study beforehand, as well as review the videotape of the study with them afterward.

N O T E S

Normal Radiographic Anatomy and Physiology of the Oropharynx

Lateral Plane

The MBS usually begins with the patient viewed in the lateral plane (Dodds, Logemann, & Stewart, 1990). This radiographic view provides the clinician with the best observation of oral and pharyngeal anatomy and physiology and of the separation of the airway and the esophagus. At some point in the radiographic study, the patient should be turned and viewed in the posterior-anterior (P-A) plane during swallows of selected bolus types, in order to determine the symmetry of the swallow. There are a number of anatomic landmarks in the head-and-neck region that facilitate identification of the structures in the upper aerodigestive tract.

Anatomy

Figure 2.1 shows a patient positioned and ready for an MBS, facing left (viewed in the lateral plane). This orientation is similar to that used in most phonetics and articulation textbooks. Oropharyngeal structures are labeled and numbered in Figure 2.2 in the order in which they are most easily identified on X ray. This represents a simple method of orientation to the radiographic anatomy of the head and neck.

The lower rim of the mandible should be identified first. The two sides of the lower rim of the mandible are often both visible in the lateral view (1–2). No head stabilization is used in the MBS, so the patient is rarely examined in a perfect midsagittal plane. If the observer's eye traces backward along the lower rim of the mandible and slightly inferiorly, the hyoid bone (3) is usually identifiable. On fluoroscopy in the lateral plane, the body of the hyoid is seen as an oval or rounded shape. The greater horns of the hyoid, which project posteriorly, are not usually visible on fluoroscopy because they are not densely ossified. Located posterior and often slightly inferior to the body of the hyoid bone is the epiglottis (4), which extends inferiorly to the thyroid notch, where it attaches via a ligament to the thyroid cartilage. If the observer's eye then moves down from the epiglottis, the entry to the airway (the laryngeal vestibule, (5) can be seen. The laryngeal vestibule is bounded by the epiglottis anteriorly, the aryepiglottic folds laterally, and the arytenoid cartilages (6) posteriorly. Inferiorly, the aryepiglottic folds terminate in the false vocal folds. Below the false vocal folds are the ventricles and the true vocal folds (7).

If the observer's eye returns to the epiglottis and moves superiorly rather than inferiorly, the vallecula (8) is located immediately behind the epiglottis. The vallecula is the space formed between the epiglottis and the base of the tongue (9). In Figure 2.2, the valleculae are filled with residual barium. The lingual tonsils are located at the

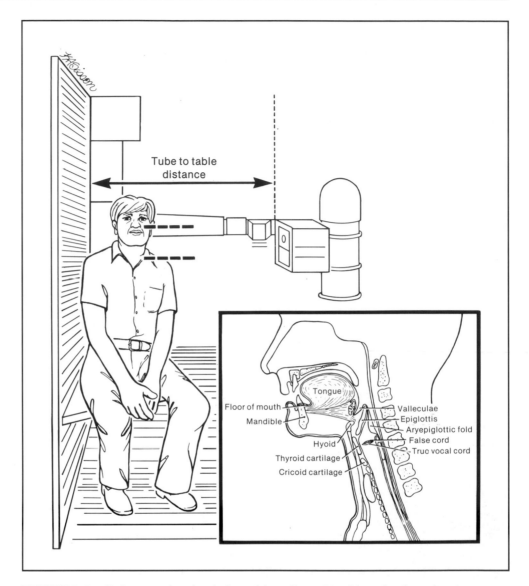

FIGURE 2.1.   Patient seated on the platform of the radiographic table so that the oral cavity, pharynx, and cervical esophagus can be viewed in the lateral plane, as shown in the lower right-hand corner.

base of the tongue. Following the base of the tongue upward, the back of the tongue becomes visible, as do the velum and the oral cavity (*10*). The back of the tongue and the base of the tongue are different anatomic areas. The base of the tongue extends from the valleculae to the circumvallate papillae (approximately at the tip of the uvula). The back of the tongue begins at the circumvallate papillae and extends to the front of the soft palate and is used to articulate /k/ and /g/.

With this orientation, the observer should be able to identify the basic structures viewed laterally in the head-and-neck region. In addition to these structures, the cervical spine should be examined for arthritic changes or for any excessive anterior bony growth (cervical osteophytes) that may impinge on the posterior pharyngeal wall and thus narrow the pharynx.

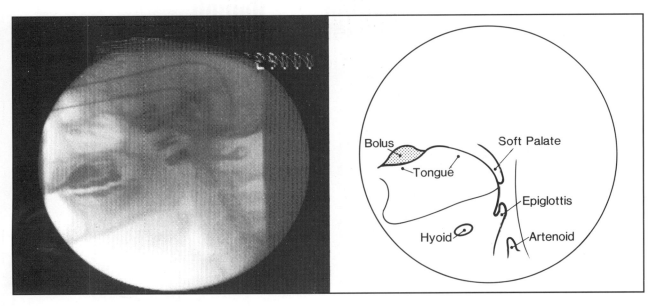

FIGURE 2.5. A lateral view (videoprint) of the initiation of the oral stage of swallow, with the tongue having picked up the bolus from the floor of the mouth.

the epiglottis is accomplished by anterior tilting of the arytenoid before the larynx begins to elevate. The mobile top third of the epiglottis is also being folded down to horizontal by the upward and forward movement of the larynx and hyoid. On larger bolus volumes, the force of the downward-moving bolus contributes to epiglottic descent (Logemann et al., 1992).

As the bolus tail approaches the top of the tongue base, contraction of the pharyngeal walls (anterior movement of the posterior pharyngeal wall and medial move-

N O T E S

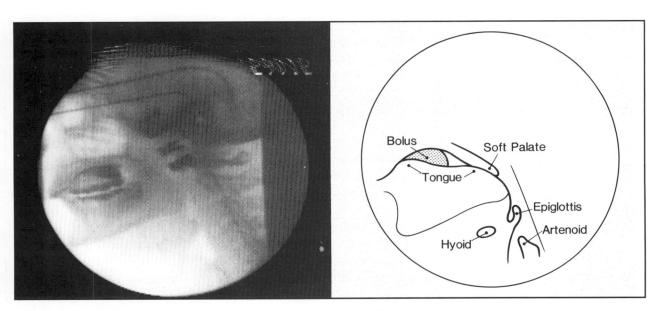

FIGURE 2.6. A lateral view (videoprint) of the head and neck illustrating the onset of oral transit, with the tongue initiating propulsion of the bolus by applying pressure to the bolus tail.

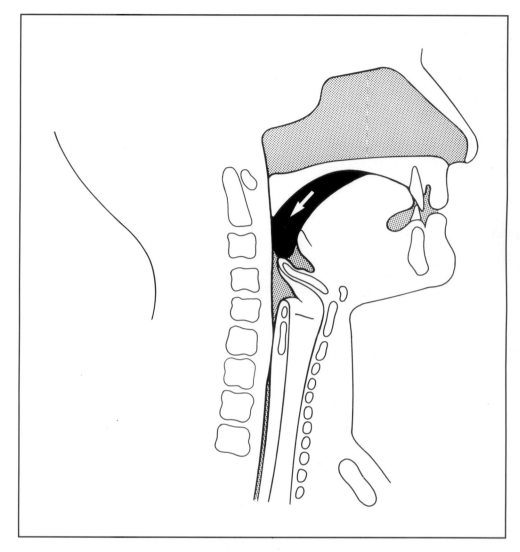

FIGURE 2.7.   A lateral view of the head and neck illustrating the transition to the pharyngeal swallow, with the oral tongue applying pressure to the tail of the bolus in the oral cavity, and the head of the bolus entering the valleculae. The pharyngeal swallow has been triggered. Velopharyngeal closure is accomplished, the larynx is in process of elevating and closing, and the upper esophageal sphincter is still closed.

ment of the lateral pharyngeal wall) begins at the oropharynx and the tongue base moves posteriorly to meet the inward-moving pharynx. The tongue base contacts the anteriorly and medially moving pharyngeal walls, which together generate pressure to continue bolus propulsion through the pharynx. Figure 2.8 illustrates a 3-ml bolus at the tongue base just before posterior motion of the tongue base and contraction of the pharyngeal walls. Figure 2.9 illustrates contact of the tongue base and posterior pharyngeal wall just above the valleculae.

Posterior movement of the tongue base and pharyngeal-wall contraction occur later in the swallow as bolus volume increases. Contraction of the pharyngeal wall progresses superiorly to inferiorly, following the bolus tail. Tongue-base movement is considered the major pressure-generating force to propel the bolus through the pharynx, while pharyngeal contraction is considered a clearing wave to clean any residual bolus from the pharyngeal walls. In the lateral view, posterior movement of the tongue base covers approximately two-thirds of the distance to the posterior pharyngeal wall, while anterior bulging of the pharynx covers one-third of the distance (Kahrilas, Logemann, Lin, & Ergun, 1992).

As the bolus head (leading edge) approaches the upper esophageal sphincter (UES) (cricopharyngeal region), the UES opens by a complex series of events, beginning with relaxation of whatever tone is present in the cricopharyngeus muscle. This is considered a facilitatory event, since relaxation of the muscle does not open the sphincter. As the hyolaryngeal complex moves up and forward, anterior movement of the cricoid cartilage (the anterior wall of the sphincter) opens the sphincter. As the bolus enters the UES, the pressure of the bolus widens the opening. Larger boluses with larger intrabolus pressure result in a wider UES opening (Cook, Dodds, Dantas,

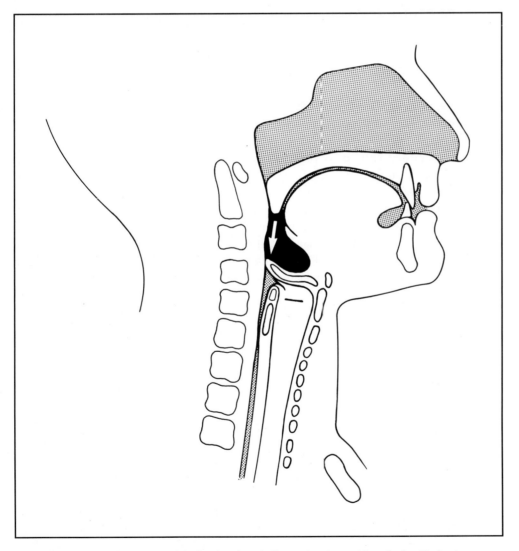

FIGURE 2.8. A lateral view of the head and neck illustrating the position of a 3-ml bolus just before posterior movement of the tongue base and pharyngeal-wall contraction.

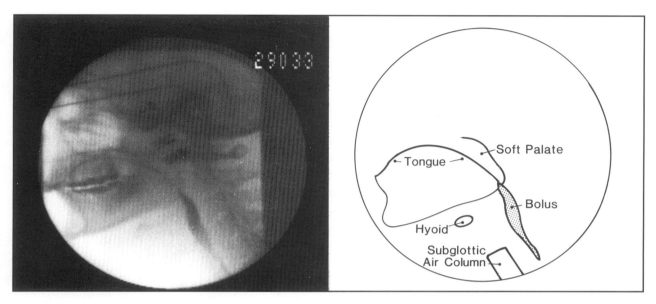

FIGURE 2.9.   A lateral view (videoprint) of the head and neck illustrating contact of the tongue base to the pharyngeal wall above the valleculae behind the bolus tail.

N O T E S

Massey, Kern, Lang, Brasseur, & Hogan, 1989; Jacob et al., 1989). The duration of both airway closure at the arytenoid to the base of the epiglottis and opening of the cricopharyngeal region is significantly prolonged as bolus volume increases. Unless the airway is closed early on a voluntary basis (see "Variations in Normal Anatomy and Physiology" later in this chapter), airway closure and UES opening generally occur within ±0.06 sec of each other (Logemann et al., 1992). The bolus head normally reaches the UES just as it opens, so that no bolus hesitation exists in the pyriform sinuses before the UES opens. Figure 2.10 illustrates bolus passage through the UES and into the cervical esophagus. After the swallow, there should be minimal residue remaining in the mouth and pharynx, as shown in Figure 2.11. Normal residue consists of a coating of material on the oral and/or pharyngeal structures rather than any significant amount of food.

For boluses requiring *chewing*, there is rotary, lateral motion of the tongue and mandible (Logemann, 1983). Tongue motion is most critical for control of the bolus, placing it onto the teeth, picking it up from the teeth, mixing it with saliva, and replacing it onto the teeth. When chewing is complete, the tongue forms a bolus of appropriate size and holds the bolus momentarily, as described earlier; then the oral swallow is initiated as described above.

During sequential *swallowing from a cup*, airway closure may be maintained as two to six swallows of 15 to 20 ml are taken sequentially with repeated tongue gestures. UES opening is not maintained throughout this interval, but reopens as each bolus approaches.

During *straw drinking*, the soft palate is usually pulled anteriorly against the back of the tongue, forming a firm seal and allowing intraoral suction to draw liquid up the straw and into the mouth. When the bolus has filled the mouth, the swallow is initiated and proceeds as described above. Thus, normally, straw drinking only affects the way in which liquid is drawn into the mouth. A second method of straw drinking is dangerous. In this technique, the patient maintains an open oropharyngeal airway

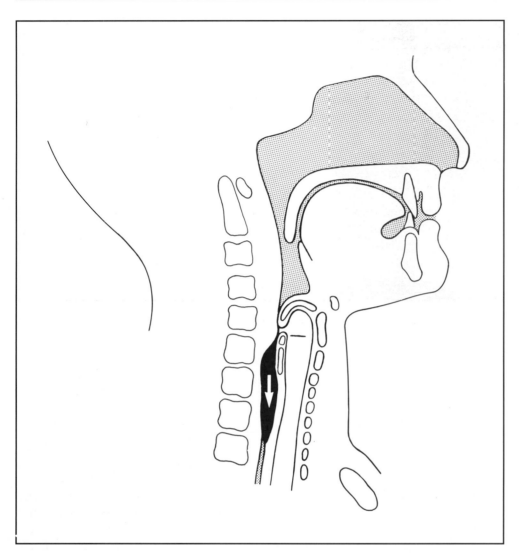

FIGURE 2.10. A lateral view of the head and neck illustrating the end of the pharyngeal swallow, with the bolus passing through the upper esophageal sphincter and into the cervical esophagus. Pharyngeal structures are in process of relaxing.

(with no soft palate descent) and uses inhalation to "suck" liquids into the mouth. This method can result in aspiration and should not be used.

Swallowing of saliva is normally only a small volume (1–2 ml). If saliva is located in the oral cavity, the swallowing sequence is similar to that described above. If the saliva is located in the pharynx, the pharyngeal swallow will activate to clear the saliva bolus with no oral-stage movement.

Posterior-Anterior Plane

Anatomy

In the P-A plane, the oral cavity and tongue can be seen, particularly the shaping of the tongue around the bolus (Figure 2.12) (Dodds, et al., 1990). The mid tongue (*1*)

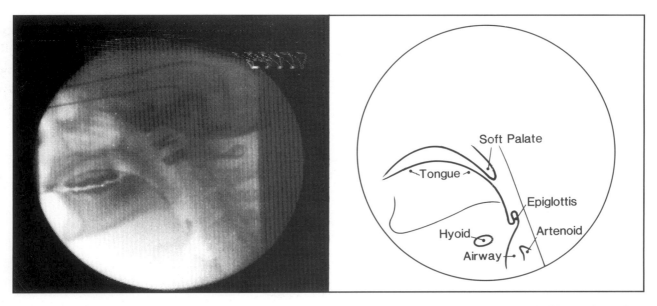

FIGURE 2.11. A lateral view (videoprint) of the oral cavity and pharynx after the swallow, with normal (negligible) residue in the mouth and pharynx.

and the sides of the tongue (*2*) are clearly visible. Looking more inferiorly, the valleculae (*3*) are seen as scalloped in shape, with the hyoepiglottic ligament (*4*) dividing the valleculae. The lateral pharyngeal walls are visible from the valleculae to the pyriform sinuses (*6*). The soft tissues of the pharynx are often not clearly visible on the P-A view unless contrast material is present. This is unlike the lateral view, in which air normally provides sufficient contrast to view the pharyngeal structures.

The contour of the larynx can also sometimes be viewed in the P-A plane, particularly if aspiration occurs. As shown in Figure 2.13, the false vocal folds, ventricle,

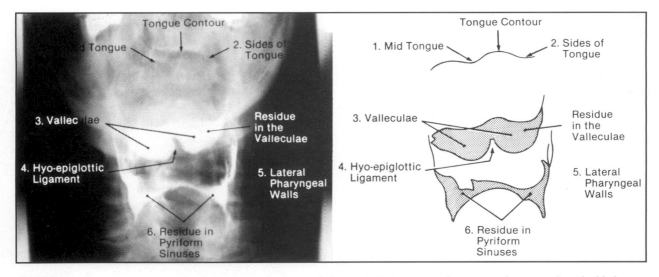

FIGURE 2.12. A posterior-anterior view of an oral cavity and pharynx containing more than a normal amount of residual bolus, which outlines the contour of the tongue orally and the valleculae and pyriform sinuses in the pharynx.

and true vocal folds can be seen. Unless aspiration occurs, these structures are most easily viewed during phonation and respiration when the patient switches between abduction (inhalation) and adduction (phonation), as discussed in Chapter 4.

Physiology

In the P-A plane, swallowing physiology appears quite different than in the lateral view. As the bolus enters the mouth, lingual shaping around the bolus with the sides elevated to the alveolar ridge is clearly visible. The lateral motions of the tongue during chewing are also easily examined. Lingual posterior propulsion of the bolus is only partially seen. As the bolus reaches the valleculae, it usually divides fairly evenly and moves laterally through the two pyriform sinuses and into the esophagus. However, in approximately 20% of normal swallows, the bolus passes down only one side. In the P-A view, medial superior-to-inferior movement of the lateral walls is dramatic, following the tail of the bolus through the pharynx.

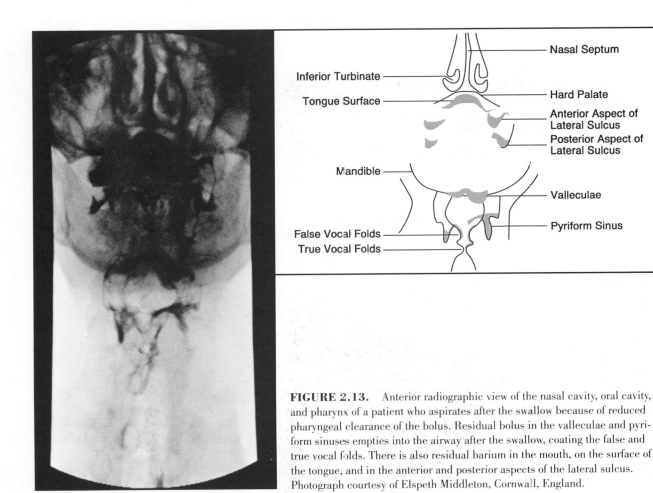

FIGURE 2.13. Anterior radiographic view of the nasal cavity, oral cavity, and pharynx of a patient who aspirates after the swallow because of reduced pharyngeal clearance of the bolus. Residual bolus in the valleculae and pyriform sinuses empties into the airway after the swallow, coating the false and true vocal folds. There is also residual barium in the mouth, on the surface of the tongue, and in the anterior and posterior aspects of the lateral sulcus. Photograph courtesy of Elspeth Middleton, Cornwall, England.

Variations in Normal Anatomy and Physiology

The normal anatomy of a young infant and child differs from that of a young adult and an older adult. After surgical ablation, radiographic anatomy of the oral cavity or pharynx may be altered. These variations are discussed and illustrated.

Infants and Young Children

In infants and young children, the anatomic relationship between the structures of the oral cavity and pharynx is different from that of adults. In the infant, the tongue fills the oral cavity, and the hyoid bone and larynx are much higher than in adults (Figure 2.14), affording more natural protection for the airway (Bosma, 1986; Newman, Cleveland, Blickman, Hillman, & Jaramillo, 1991). The velum usually hangs lower, with the uvula often resting inside the epiglottis, forming a pocket in the valleculae. As described below, the bolus often is collected in the vallecular pocket with repeated tongue pumps. During facial growth, the jaw grows down and forward, carrying the tongue down and enlarging the oral cavity space between the tongue and palate. The larynx lowers as does the hyoid bone, thereby enlarging the pharynx. The greatest elongation of the pharynx and downward displacement of the larynx occurs during puberty.

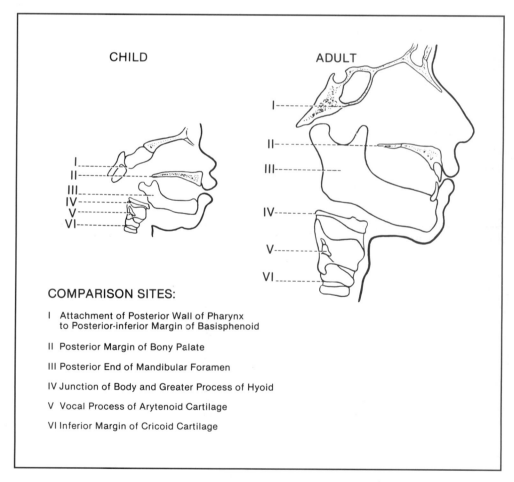

CHILD

ADULT

COMPARISON SITES:

I   Attachment of Posterior Wall of Pharynx
    to Posterior-inferior Margin of Basisphenoid

II Posterior Margin of Bony Palate

III Posterior End of Mandibular Foramen

IV Junction of Body and Greater Process of Hyoid

V Vocal Process of Arytenoid Cartilage

VI Inferior Margin of Cricoid Cartilage

FIGURE 2.14.   Lateral drawings of the bony and cartilaginous structures of the oral cavity and larynx in the child and the adult, illustrating the comparative positioning of the mandible and laryngeal cartilages.

Swallowing physiology in the infant is quite different from that of the adult. When sucking from a nipple, the infant repeatedly pumps the tongue, expressing milk from the nipple with each pump and collecting this liquid at the faucial arches (in front of the anteriorly bulging soft palate) or in the valleculae. Each infant tends to follow a pattern of using a particular number of tongue pumps predominantly, with some variability. Normal infants may use anywhere from two to seven tongue pumps (Newman et al., 1991). More than that would be considered abnormal. Usually the number of tongue pumps used relates to the amount of liquid expressed from the nipple by a single tongue movement, that is, fewer tongue motions if a large amount of liquid is expressed with each tongue movement, more tongue pumps if less liquid is expressed. When a bolus of adequate size has been formed, the pharyngeal swallow is triggered. The pharyngeal swallow in the infant is similar to that of the adult with two exceptions. First, laryngeal elevation is much reduced, since the larynx is anatomically elevated under the tongue base and does not need to move upward, and second, in normal infants, the posterior pharyngeal wall is often seen to move much farther anteriorly during the swallow than is observed in adults.

Older Adults

With age, ossification in the thyroid and cricoid cartilages and the hyoid bone increases, so that these structures may appear more prominent during fluoroscopy. Also, as adults reach age 70 and beyond, the larynx may begin to lower slightly in the neck, approaching the seventh cervical vertebra. With age, the incidence of cervical arthritis increases. Arthritic changes in the cervical vertebrae may impinge on the pharyngeal wall, decreasing its flexibility.

Some minimal changes in oropharyngeal swallowing physiology have been noted in normal individuals over age 60 (Logemann, 1990a; Robbins, Hamilton, Lof, & Kempster, 1992; Sonies, Baum, & Shawker, 1984; Tracy et al., 1989). Older individuals more frequently hold the bolus on the floor of the mouth and pick it up with the tongue tip as the oral stage of swallowing is initiated (Dodds et al., 1989). The oral stage of swallowing is slightly longer in older adults as is the "normal" delay in triggering the pharyngeal swallow (Figure 2.15). These differences are of small magnitude (less than a second).

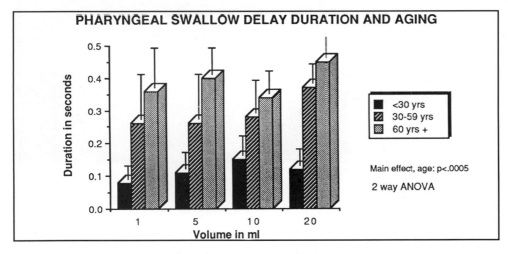

FIGURE 2.15. A bar graph illustrating the mean and standard error for pharyngeal swallow delay in three groups of normal subjects. Normal older subjects over age 60 exhibit a statistically significantly longer delay in triggering the pharyngeal swallow than young adults.

No increase has been observed in frequency or extent of oral or pharyngeal residue, penetration of material into the laryngeal vestibule, or aspiration in older adults. Figure 2.16 illustrates the range of pharyngeal residue (least to most) observed in older subjects in our studies. This figure can serve as a reference for normal residue versus abnormal pharyngeal residue observed in older dysphagic subjects.

In contrast to the small changes in oropharyngeal swallowing physiology in older adults, esophageal function deteriorates more significantly with age so that esophageal transit and clearance are slower and less efficient after age 70 (Mandelstam & Lieber, 1970).

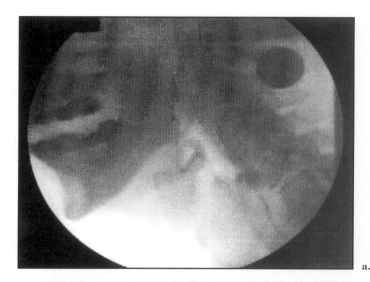

a.

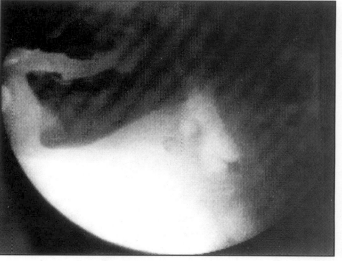

b.

FIGURE 2.16.
(*a*) A lateral view (video-print) of the oral cavity and pharynx of an 87-year-old adult after the swallow, illustrating the maximal amount of residue observed in normal elderly subjects. There is a small amount of residue in the valleculae and pyriform sinuses.
(*b*) A lateral view (video-print) of the oral cavity and pharynx of an 83-year-old adult after the swallow, illustrating the least amount of residue observed in normal elderly subjects. There is a light coating on the tongue and the pyriform sinuses.

Head-and-Neck Surgical Patients

Surgical procedures for head-and-neck cancer often result in changes in radiographic anatomy, in either the lateral or anterior-posterior plane. The most common surgical procedures and the changes they effect in anatomy are discussed in the following paragraphs.

Oral cancer procedures. A wide variety of ablative surgical procedures for cancer of the oral cavity can result in anatomic changes in oral structure, particularly in the mandible, tongue, and soft palate (Logemann, 1983, 1985, 1990b). In the lateral radiographic view, a partial mandibulectomy can usually be seen (Figure 2.17) if the patient is not positioned in a perfect midsagittal view.

Resection of portions of the anterior tongue or tongue base may also be clearly visible in the lateral plane, especially after several swallows when oral structures are coated with barium (Figure 2.18). Reduction in tissue on the lateral margin of the tongue will usually be seen in the lateral view only as food collects on the tongue or in the enlarged lateral floor of the mouth (Figure 2.19). In the P-A view, the absence of lateral tongue tissue can be observed as the patient attempts to hold the bolus or during oral transit.

To better understand the patterns of oral function seen during radiographic studies of oral transit of material in these oral cancer patients, the clinician should complete a careful oral examination, identifying the limits of the surgical resection, the nature of the reconstruction, the location of suture lines, and new relationships

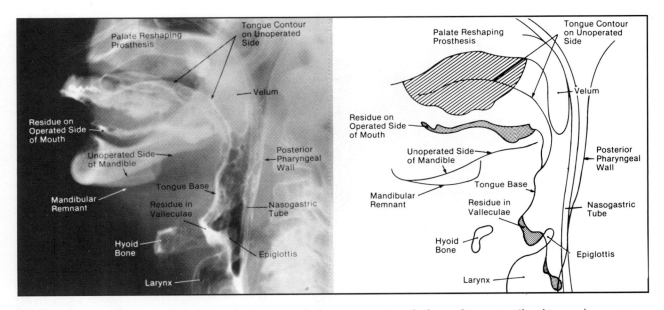

FIGURE 2.17. A lateral radiograph of the oral cavity and pharynx in a patient who has undergone tonsil and tongue-base resection with partial mandibulectomy. Residual food on the operated side of the oral cavity can be seen, as can mild residual food in the valleculae and pyriform sinus. The patient is wearing a palate-lowering or reshaping prosthesis, which can also be seen.

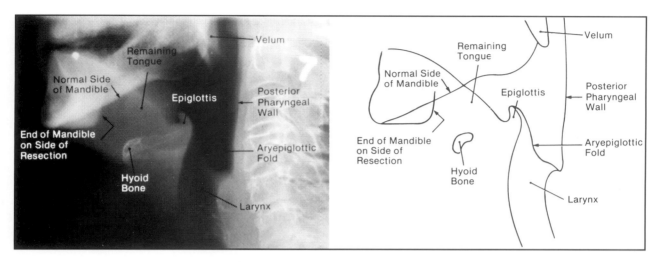

FIGURE 2.18. A lateral view of the oral cavity and pharynx in a patient who has undergone tonsil and tongue-base resection with partial mandibulectomy. The abnormal shape of the remaining posterior tongue and tongue base is clearly visible.

N O T E S   between oral structures *before* the radiographic procedure (MBS) is begun. This facilitates interpretation of the radiographic anatomy and physiology.

   Hemilaryngectomy. The hemilaryngectomy procedure removes one vertical half of the larynx including a part of the thyroid cartilage, one false vocal fold, one ventricle, and one true vocal fold on the same side (usually excluding the arytenoid cartilage). The hyoid bone and epiglottis are usually spared. Variations on the hemi-

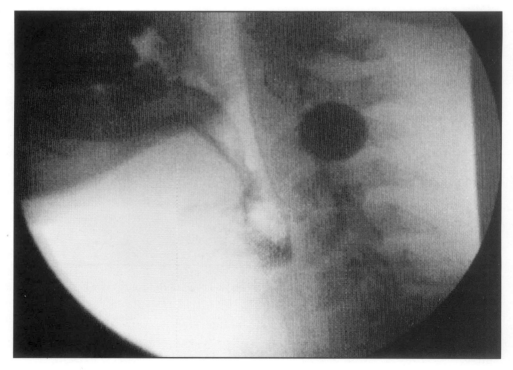

FIGURE 2.19. A lateral view of the oral cavity and pharynx illustrating asymmetry in the two sides of the oral tongue and tongue base, which are each coated with barium.

laryngectomy procedure include extension around the anterior commissure, removing part of the other vocal fold anteriorly and/or laterally, or posterior extension to include part or all of the arytenoid. The location of the tumor dictates the exact limits of the resection. In the lateral radiographic plane, there are usually no visible changes in radiographic anatomy in the hemilaryngectomee. In the P-A plane, the laryngeal contours are normal on one side and are replaced or reconstructed on the opposite side by soft tissue (usually part of one of the strap muscles). When examining such a patient radiographically, it is important to note whether the reconstructed mass on the side of the resection corresponds in height to the normal side of the larynx, particularly to the vocal fold, so that the patient can accomplish closure of the airway during the swallow by approximation of the normal vocal fold against the reconstructed tissue.

Prior to radiographic examination of the hemilaryngectomized patient, the clinician should determine the exact extent of the patient's surgical resection and the nature of the reconstruction, since there are many variations on this surgical procedure that may affect the patient's swallowing ability and duration of recovery to normal swallowing (Rademaker et al., in press).

Supraglottic laryngectomy.   The supraglottic laryngectomy procedure removes the top two sphincters of the airway: the epiglottis and aryepiglottic folds and the false vocal folds (McConnel et al., 1987; Sessions, Zil, & Schwartz, 1979). The hyoid bone and a small part of the base of the tongue may be included in the resection. The arytenoid cartilages and true vocal folds are usually spared, though a part of the arytenoid is occasionally resected if the supraglottic surgery is extended inferiorly. In the lateral radiographic view, the base of the tongue ends at the true vocal folds (Fig. 2.20). The epiglottis and hyoid bone are absent.

During the swallow, the arytenoids and tongue base will make contact, closing the entry to the airway and preventing aspiration. This closure of the reconstructed laryngeal entrance is learned after surgery and can be practiced with the supersupraglottic swallow (Chapter 4). A second, less frequent method of airway protection during the swallow in these patients involves closure of the true vocal folds. Food or liquid will be seen to reach the true vocal folds and then to be squeezed clear of the larynx, as the larynx lifts and closes at the arytenoid-to-tongue-base level. If the larynx fails to lift or close at the arytenoid level during the swallow, material sitting above the vocal folds must be coughed clear or it will be aspirated after the swallow.

In the P-A view, the normal laryngeal contour is changed so that only the true vocal folds are present and the false vocal folds and ventricle are removed. Movement of the two vocal folds should be carefully assessed in the P-A plane to determine the patient's ability to approximate the folds during the swallow.

Total laryngectomy.   A total laryngectomy removes the entire larynx, from and including the hyoid bone and a small amount of tongue base superiorly to below the cricoid cartilage inferiorly. The airway (tracheal stump) is then brought forward and sutured to the outside skin of the lower neck to form a stoma. The airway is therefore permanently separated from the pharynx and esophagus. The pharynx and esophagus are reconstructed into a single tube, the pharyngoesophagus, and the base of the tongue connects directly to the pharynx. Usually, there is no longer any identifiable anatomic boundary between the pharynx and the esophagus. The contraction within the pharynx and the peristalsis in the cervical esophagus are often reduced, less coordinated, or absent, so that tongue propulsion and gravity carry the food or liquid into the body of the esophagus. The total laryngectomee may exhibit repeated tongue movements in order to compensate for reduced pharyngeal coordination by increased

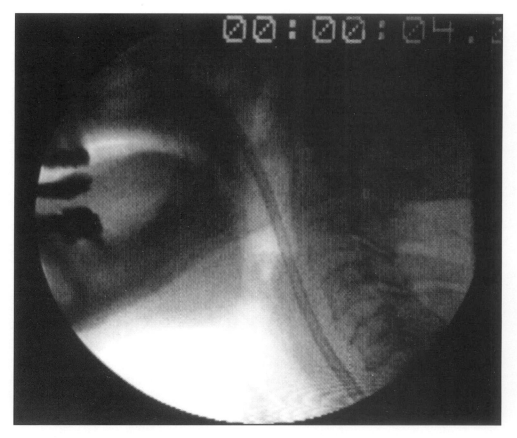

FIGURE 2.20. A lateral radiographic videoprint of a supraglottic laryngectomee with a nasogastric tube in place. The patient's epiglottis, hyoid bone, aryepiglottic folds, and false vocal folds have been removed, leaving the tongue base and arytenoid cartilage constituting the reconstructed airway entrance.

tongue pressure and activity (McConnel et al., 1986; McConnel, Hester, Mendelsohn, & Logemann, 1988). Also, with hyoid bone removal, the foundation for the tongue is gone, thus affecting its fine-coordination ability.

A pseudoepiglottis may be seen in some total laryngectomees (Figure 2.21). This fold of soft tissue is situated at the tongue base and often looks like an epiglottis. If it is small and asymptomatic, as in Figure 2.21, it will not interfere with the swallow. If it is large, it can form a pocket where food collects.

Total laryngectomy, pharyngectomy, and esophagectomy reconstructed by gastric pull-up. This procedure uses the stomach to reconstruct a large surgical defect, that is, removal of the entire larynx, pharynx, and esophagus. The stomach is loosened from its lower attachments in the abdominal cavity and is stretched up and sutured directly to the base of the tongue (Fig. 2.22). As a result of this procedure, there is no peristaltic action to bring the food to the stomach. Rather, food is propelled from the mouth by the tongue and falls over the back of the tongue and down into the stomach. Successive swallows push one bolus after another farther into the stomach by gravity. After approximately one hour, the stomach empties. Patients who have had such reconstruction must usually remain upright after eating so that food does not backflow into the mouth, as there is no valve at the top of the stomach and base of the tongue to

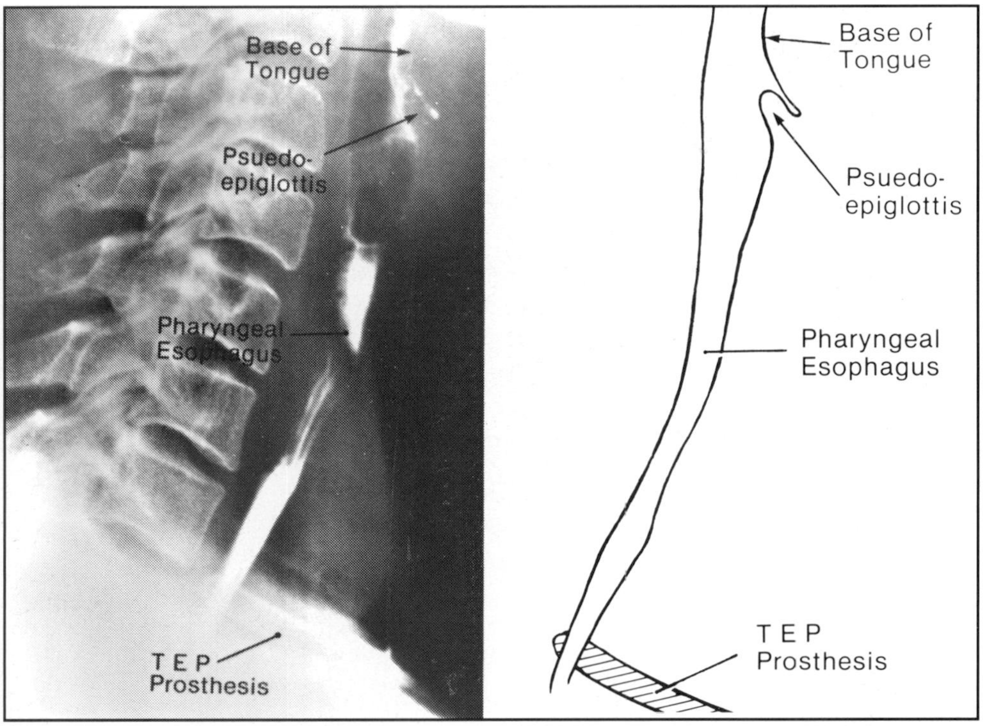

FIGURE 2.21.   A lateral radiographic view of a total laryngectomee's pharyngoesophagus with an asymptomatic pseudoepiglottis identified. The patient is wearing a tracheoesophageal puncture (TEP) prosthesis at the base of the cervical esophagus.

prevent this reflux. Radiographically, the stretched and elongated stomach often resembles the esophagus.

Variations in Normal and Abnormal Oropharyngeal Physiology

Changes in Timing of the Oral and Pharyngeal Phases— Bolus Volume Effect

During swallows of small boluses (1 to 3 ml) including saliva, the oral phase of swallowing is followed by the pharyngeal phase and then the esophageal phase. On swallows of larger bolus volumes (5 to 20 ml), the oral and pharyngeal phases of swallowing increasingly overlap, until on 20-ml boluses, the oral and pharyngeal phases occur simultaneously. These changes are systematic and predictable in normal swallowers to accommodate the increasing bolus volume.

In addition, the duration of pharyngeal swallow events changes systematically with larger bolus volumes. As volume increases, the airway remains closed longer, the cricopharyngeal region opens longer and wider, and the hyoid bone remains elevated longer (Cook, Dodds, Dantas, Kern, Massey, Shaker, & Hogan, 1989; Dantas et al., 1990; Dodds et al., 1975; Dodds et al., 1988; Jacob et al., 1989; Kahrilas, Dodds, Dent, Logemann, & Shaker, 1988; Kahrilas, Lin, Logemann, Ergun, & Facchini, in press; Logemann et al., 1992).

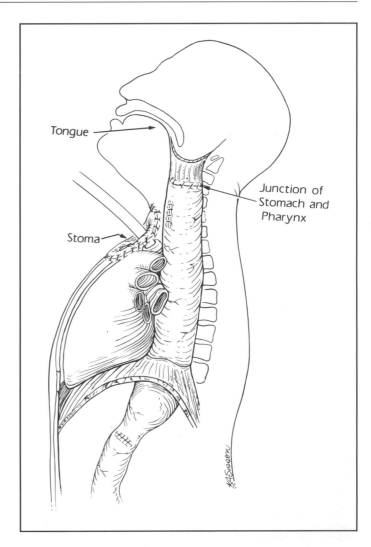

FIGURE 2.22. The reconstructed anatomy of a total laryngectomee-esophagectomee with stomach pull-up. The stomach is freed from the ligaments in the abdomen and stretched to anastomose at the tongue base.

Changes in Timing of the Oral and Pharyngeal Phases— Bolus Viscosity Effect

With more viscous boluses, there is prolongation of oral and pharyngeal transit times and increased width of cricopharyngeal opening. Lingual pressure used to propel the bolus through the oral cavity increases as bolus viscosity increases (Dantas, Dodds, Massey, & Kern, 1989).

Because of these systematic changes in oropharyngeal swallowing physiology as bolus volume and viscosity increase, it is important to determine the patient's ability to manage these adjustments. The radiographic study should include boluses calibrated for various volumes and several viscosities.

Protective Behaviors

Some normal individuals, as well as patients who have experienced swallowing difficulties, learn to protect their pharynx by producing one of several gestures. Some patients will bring food back from their pharynx after a swallowing attempt. These patients initiate the oral swallow and propel the bolus down to the pyriform sinus; wait for a pharyngeal swallow; and, when one is delayed, bring the food back into the oral cavity. This is done with a backward gesture of the tongue base and a forward squeezing of the pharyngeal wall (Figure 2.23). Other patients will initiate the oral swallow and propel food back to the vallecular level. When the food reaches the valleculae, these patients bring it immediately back into the mouth. This behavior protects the pharynx by not allowing food to remain there long enough to be aspirated.

Some normal and dysphagic individuals close their airway early, especially in response to larger bolus volumes. On 10-ml liquid boluses or cup drinking, these individuals close the airway at the arytenoid-to-base-of-epiglottis level before the swallow begins and maintain that closure throughout the swallow. On lateral radiographic view during these swallows, the arytenoid cartilage can be observed to tilt anteriorly to contact the base of the epiglottis before laryngeal elevation begins.

Compensatory Behaviors

Some dysphagic patients will spontaneously vary their head position to assist their swallowing. The two most commonly used head movements are tossing the head backward to assist oral clearance by gravity, or tilting the head downward to facilitate contact between the tongue base and the pharyngeal wall and improved pharyngeal clearance of the bolus.

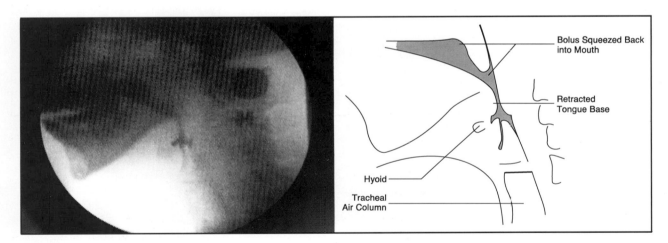

FIGURE 2.23.   A lateral videoprint of a voluntary maneuver to bring food from the pharynx and back into the oral cavity. The tongue base is retracted and the pharyngeal wall is contracted at the tongue-base level, squeezing against the food to bring it back into the mouth and thus protecting the airway from aspiration.

N O T E S

Modified Barium Swallow Procedure

Rationale for the Modified Barium Swallow Procedure

The modified barium swallow (MBS) procedure is designed to study the anatomy and the physiology of the oral preparatory, oral, pharyngeal, and cervical esophageal stages of deglutition (Logemann, 1983) and to define management and treatment strategies that will improve the oropharyngeal dysphagic patient's swallowing safety or efficiency. The problems encountered in the radiographic assessment of these aspects of swallowing are very different from those experienced during fluoroscopic examination of the esophageal stage of deglutition (Dodds, Logemann, & Stewart, 1990; Dodds et al., 1990). Thus, the MBS procedure, as described here, is needed to assess patients with oral or pharyngeal dysphagia, and a barium swallow procedure is needed to examine esophageal anatomy and physiology. The two procedures should not be combined into a single assessment. A patient who needs both assessments should receive an MBS first, followed by an esophageal assessment, once it is determined that the patient can tolerate the larger volume of barium used in the esophageal evaluation.

Because the esophagus is a collapsed muscular tube, a larger bolus is needed in order to distend the esophagus and define its outline and contour and to see and assess the peristaltic wave during the swallow. Thus, in the standard barium swallow procedure, the patient is given a cup of barium and asked to continue to swallow until told to stop. Because esophageal peristalsis is being assessed, the patient is often examined while lying down and is viewed in the P-A plane. In this position, gravity is eliminated and the bolus moves primarily because of esophageal peristaltic action (Dodds, Hogan, Reid, Stewart, & Arndorfer, 1973).

In contrast to the esophagus, the oral cavity and pharynx, by definition, are cavities. They do not need to be filled with barium or with other radiopaque substances in order for the clinician to identify the outline of the structures or their movement. In fact, when the oral cavity and pharynx are filled with radiopaque material, the structures are partially obliterated, as is their physiology. Thus, in an MBS procedure, the patient is initially given a very small amount of material to swallow (1 ml—equivalent to approximately ⅓ teaspoon) so that the anatomy and physiology of the oral cavity and pharynx can be viewed accurately. Then, bolus volume is slowly and systematically increased, as tolerated. Also, because patients with swallowing disorders may complain of difficulty with one food consistency and not another, the patient is given food of at least three different consistencies in the process of a single study. Usually these include a liquid, a paste or puddinglike material (usually Esophatrast mixed with pudding), and something requiring mastication, usually a cookie. In all cases, only a small amount of material is used initially, generally 1 ml, followed by 3 ml, 5 ml, and

10 ml of the liquid and cup drinking of the liquid, if tolerated; ⅓ teaspoon of the pudding material; and one-quarter of an easily chewed shortbread cookie.

A second reason for initially limiting the amount of material presented, and increasing it systematically as tolerated, is the potential for aspiration. Many of the patients sent for an MBS are at risk of significant aspiration or are known aspirators, possibly with chronic obstructive pulmonary disease, aspiration pneumonia, or other pulmonary complications. In these cases, the patient's attending physician is normally concerned about the patient aspirating a significant amount of material during the radiographic procedure. Therefore, it is important to place the patient at minimal risk for aspiration by providing him or her with a small amount of material. Larger amounts of liquid per bolus are presented as tolerated. However, this is never done in the first several swallows.

Finally, in contrast to the traditional barium swallow, during the MBS patients are viewed initially in their normal eating position, usually upright and in the lateral plane. Since gravity plays a role in moving the bolus through the pharynx in normal deglutition, it is this effect of gravity in the normal position that must be assessed. A lateral plane is used to examine two important aspects of the swallow that are the most visible and measurable in the lateral view: the speed of the swallow (i.e., oral and pharyngeal transit times) and the approximate amount of the bolus that may be aspirated (i.e., enter into the airway below the level of the true vocal folds).

After each swallow, the oral cavity and pharynx should be kept in view rather than following the bolus into the esophagus. Many patients aspirate after the swallow (Lazarus & Logemann, 1987; Veis & Logemann, 1985). This type of aspiration will be missed if the fluoroscopic tube follows the bolus into the esophagus. It is also important to note whether the patient coughs in response to any aspiration, indicating normal laryngeal sensation, and whether this cough is productive, that is, successfully eliminating the aspirated material from the airway. Residue in the pharynx after the swallow is another common sequela of dysphagia. It is significant to note whether the patient dry swallows to clear this residue, indicating normal pharyngeal sensation.

In summary, the MBS is designed to (a) examine the anatomy and physiology of the oral cavity and pharynx during deglutition, (b) identify the disorders in movement patterns of oropharyngeal structures that control the bolus and cause aspiration or inefficient swallowing (residue), and (c) define treatment strategies that will eliminate aspiration and/or increase swallow efficiency. Many of the patients who will be examined with this procedure are at risk of significant amounts of aspiration and of the medical problems associated with the entry of material into the airway. The purposes of the study dictate the details of the procedure, which are different from the standard barium swallow procedure in a number of ways. It cannot be stressed too strongly that a standard barium swallow procedure does not provide the same information as an MBS and can put the oral-pharyngeal dysphagic patient at risk for excessive aspiration without generating the necessary information on oral, pharyngeal, and laryngeal physiology needed for accurate and effective planning of treatment.

Equipment for the Radiographic Study

The MBS procedure employs fluoroscopy, which is a radiographic technique permitting observation of movement. All fluoroscopy machines include four major parts: a table on which the patient lies or leans and that presents the X ray, a fluoroscopy tube that picks up the X ray, a monitor on which the radiographic picture is viewed, and a control room. Figure 3.1 illustrates three of these four components of the fluoroscopy equipment. The fluoroscopy image can be recorded permanently in several ways. The first is *cinefluoroscopy,* in which the image is recorded on motion picture film. The advantages of cinefluoroscopy are (a) the ability to record 60 frames/sec or more, allowing detailed slow-motion analysis of the radiographic image at a rate of ⅟₆₀ sec or more, and (b) a slightly sharper image than is available on videotape. The disadvantages of cinefluoroscopy are (a) significantly increased radiation exposure to the patient because increased radiation is needed to expose the motion picture film, (b) difficulty in recording sound on the motion picture film, so that the clinician's directions to the patient, the radiologist's comments, and other discussion conducted during the fluoroscopy study are not easily recorded, and (c) time and cost of developing film.

A second method of permanently recording the fluoroscopic image uses *videotape.* There are a number of advantages to recording the fluoroscopic image on videotape: (a) radiation exposure is significantly less than for cinefluorography; (b) the videotape can be played back immediately after recording, unlike motion picture film, which requires developing; (c) videotape is usually cheaper than motion picture film, which requires not only the purchase of the film but developing; (d) the radiographic studies of 10 to 20 patients can be recorded on one tape; (e) videotape allows real-time voice recording by simply attaching a microphone to the videocassette recorder (VCR) and positioning the microphone so that it picks up the voices of the

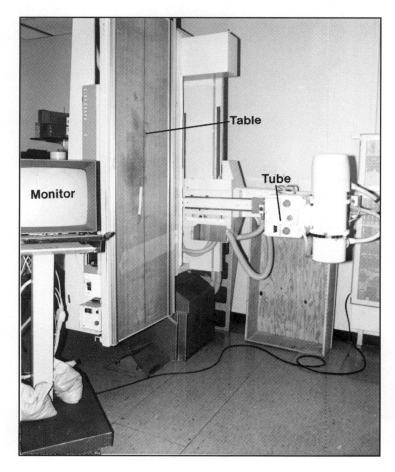

FIGURE 3.1. The fluoroscopic equipment, including the table, tube, and monitor.

examiners and the patient. A disadvantage of videotape is its usual maximum field rate of 60 fields/sec (two fields of video equals one frame), which is slower than the motion picture film speed that can be used in cinefluoroscopy. However, because swallowing is a slower function than speech, 60 fields/sec generally provides all of the detail necessary for slow-motion analysis. A second disadvantage of videotape is the slightly grainy quality of the radiographic image compared to the cinefluorographic picture.

Despite the slightly reduced image resolution of videotape (which is improving with new high-resolution systems), most clinicians and researchers are using videotape to record fluorographic studies because of the significantly reduced radiation exposure.

When recording the radiographic image on videotape, the VCR is usually attached by cable into the rear of the fluoroscopy monitor, as illustrated in Figure 3.2. In some cases, the VCR can be wired into the controls of the fluoroscopy machine so that the operator of the fluoroscopy equipment can activate the VCR and the fluoroscopy machine simultaneously. This saves videotape because the recorder is not running before and after the study. However, this latter arrangement may require more costly installation than the simple purchase of a cable to attach a VCR to the monitor.

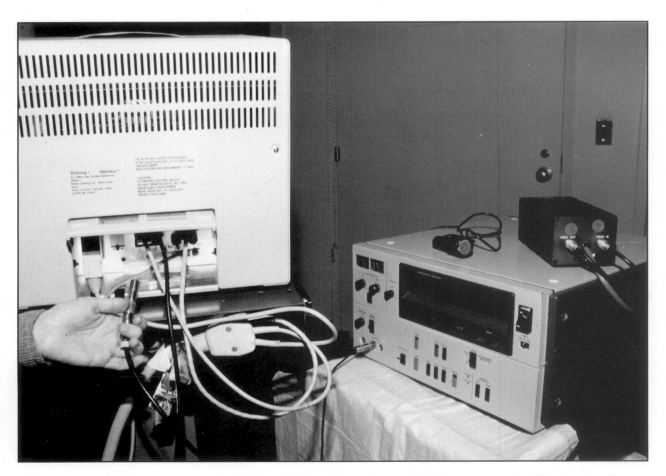

FIGURE 3.2. The videocassette recorder (VCR) attached by cable into the rear of the fluoroscopy monitor. Note the microphone sitting on top of the recorder. A counter timer is also sitting on the VCR. It encodes timing information on each field of the videotape.

In most cases, then, recording the MBS on videotape does not require a large expenditure for equipment and allows the clinician to go back and reanalyze the study repeatedly, as well as to keep the study in order to compare it with future procedures on the same patient. All that is needed is the cable to make the necessary hookup between the fluoroscopy monitor and whatever VCR the hospital has available. Almost any recorder can be used to record the image from fluoroscopy, so there is no need to purchase a special VCR unless the equipment is to be used for research purposes. However, if there is an opportunity to purchase a VCR to use in the MBS procedure, a recorder capable of easy frame-by-frame advance, variable-speed forward and reverse viewing of the tape, and stable single-frame viewing is preferable.

When the fluoroscopic study of swallowing is recorded on videotape, the clinician can use the patient's videotape for a number of teaching activities, including education of health care professionals regarding swallowing problems and education of patients and their families regarding the exact nature of the patients' swallowing problems, which may not be visible at their bedside. Because many dysphagic patients are "silent aspirators" who give no external signs of swallowing difficulty, it is easy to understand why family members continue to feed or sneak food to them despite orders from the physician or swallowing therapist not to do so. Seeing the swallowing problems on X ray increases family and patient compliance with nonoral feeding and other swallowing instructions. Similarly, nurses, dieticians, and other health professionals are often helped in their understanding of a particular patient's swallowing disorders and management strategies by watching the patient's videofluoroscopic studies.

Accessory Equipment

If the videotapes of the fluoroscopic studies are to be used for research and frame-by-frame analysis is to be completed, several additional pieces of equipment are helpful. First, a *video counter timer* can be purchased and attached to the VCR to encode numbers on the videotape at the rate of 30 or 60 per second. In this way each frame or field of the videotape is numbered. The clinician can then easily locate a particular frame for analysis and can return to the same point at any time, as desired. In order to analyze a videotape frame by frame, a VCR with high-resolution frame-pause, slow-motion forward and reverse, and single-frame advance capability is also required.

A counter timer is also useful clinically if timing of various aspects of the swallow is to be done (see Chapter 6). For example, timing information imprinted on each video frame makes measurement of the duration of pharyngeal swallow delay, airway closure, or cricopharyngeal opening quite easy.

A *video character generator* is also helpful. A character generator permits printing of the patient's name, date, and swallowing condition on the video image. In this way, each part of the videotape can be clearly labeled, and specific studies or conditions can be easily located. The character generator also prevents confusion in identification of particular swallowing interventions that are introduced.

A *video printer* produces a hard copy of a select video frame. Often rapid events or anatomic abnormalities such as fistulae are visualized only briefly during the swallowing study. A still radiograph cannot capture these rapid events. A videoprint can be made of individual video frames as they are held in frame-pause mode on a video monitor. These videoprints can then be entered into the patient's chart or sent with a report to the referring physician or other professional as a permanent representation of the disorder. A number of the figures included in this book are videoprints and are so indicated.

Standard Procedure for the Modified Barium Swallow

Though there will always be variations on the MBS procedure, as described in Chapter 4, a standard protocol of measured bolus volumes and consistencies should be used wherever and whenever possible.

Positioning the Patient

The radiographic procedure known as the modified barium swallow, rehabilitation swallow, or "cookie swallow" begins with positioning the patient in his or her usual eating position. Limitations in the design of the fluoroscopy equipment can sometimes make this difficult if the patient is unable to stand or sit unsupported. The fluoroscopic tube, which is attached to the table of the machine by an arm, often has restrictions on its range of movement, either vertically or horizontally. In many cases the maximum horizontal space between the tube and the table (only 18 to 20 in.) is not wide enough for a wheelchair. Also, the fluoroscopic tube often does not move close enough to the ground in the vertical direction to allow the operator to view the oral cavity and pharynx of a patient who is seated in a wheelchair. A number of specific chairs have been developed to facilitate the positioning of neurologically impaired patients who have poor sitting balance. These are listed in Appendix A of this book. Some fluoroscopy machines have a sufficient distance between the tube and the table to allow a cart or gurney to be positioned between them (Figure 3.3). In this case, a patient can lie on the cart with the head of the cart elevated as much as possible, to a maximum of 90°, and can be viewed laterally while lying on the cart without his or her cooperation or assistance in positioning.

If the cart is too wide to fit between the tube and table, a narrow back support can be built and used. The patient can be brought to the radiographic suite lying on the cart and can then sit up on the cart while the narrow back support is put in place. Since the back support is only 18 in. wide, the cart will slide under the tube and the back support and patient will fit between the tube and the table. If the tube-to-table distance is wide enough to accommodate a wheelchair, but the tube cannot be lowered enough to visualize the pharynx, a two-piece ramp can be constructed so that a patient seated in a wheelchair can be rolled up the ramp and positioned high enough to be viewed (Figure 3.4). Additional suggestions for positioning children are discussed in Chapter 4.

If the MBS is just being established as a procedure, the clinicians planning to use the procedure should examine the available fluoroscopy equipment to identify its limitations prior to scheduling any nonambulatory patients for the MBS. It is important to anticipate any problems with positioning patients *before bringing the patient down to X Ray,* as correcting these problems can take a great deal of time in the fluoroscopy room prior to completing the study. There usually are ways to position patients so that the study can be accomplished, if preparations are made in advance.

Supplies

A standard set of supplies should always be available in fluoroscopy. Many clinicians store supplies in the cart on which the video equipment is kept and bring both

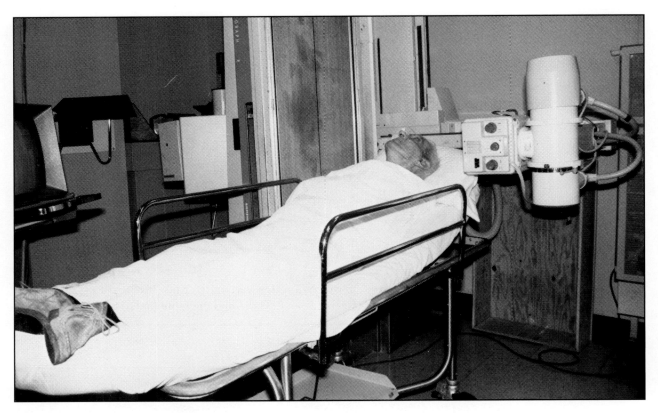

FIGURE 3.3.   The positioning of a patient on a cart. The head of the cart can be elevated to any angle from horizontal to 90° from horizontal during the radiographic study.

the cart and the supplies to Radiology when radiographic studies are scheduled. Supplies should include liquid barium, pudding barium (Esophatrast), chocolate pudding (to mix with the pudding barium), shortbread cookies, and other nonperishable foods for use in the study. The viscosities of these materials should be consistent from one study to the next. The following items should also be available: disposable plastic 1- and 10-ml syringes (minus needles), disposable plastic spoons, Mothercare spoons for patients with a bite reflex, disposable cups, tongue blades, straws, disposable gloves, measuring cups, facial tissues, and 4-by-4-in. gauze pads. Special foods or other supplies needed for a particular patient can be brought to X Ray on the day that patient is scheduled for the MBS.

Initial Radiographic Observations

Bony and soft tissue anatomy.   When the patient is positioned upright and viewed in the lateral plane, the structures in Figure 3.5 should be clearly visible. That is, the fluoroscopy tube should be focused so that the following structures are in view: the lips anteriorly, the soft palate superiorly, the posterior pharyngeal wall posteriorly, and the seventh cervical vertebrae inferiorly. In this way, the oral preparatory, oral, pharyngeal, and cervical esophageal stages of deglutition can be assessed. If all of these structures cannot be viewed simultaneously, the base of the tongue, pharynx, larynx, pyriform sinuses, and upper esophageal sphincter should be viewed first during swallows. After any disorders in the pharyngeal stage of deglutition are defined,

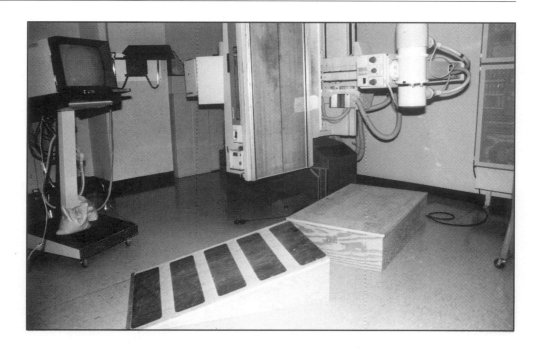

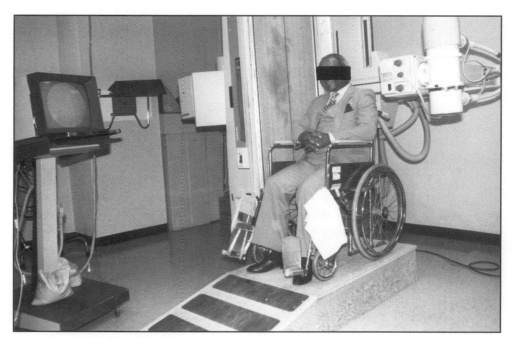

FIGURE 3.4. The plywood ramp and platform that attach to enable positioning of a wheelchair patient.

the oral cavity can be examined during several additional swallows. With the oropharyngeal structures in view, the cervical vertebrae should be examined briefly for any arthritic or other bony abnormalities such as osteophytes, which may project forward against the pharyngeal wall.

Abnormal movement patterns at rest. When the oral cavity and pharynx are in view, the position and movements of structures of the mouth and pharynx should be observed at rest for several seconds to identify any tremors, myoclonus, or other movement disorders. Myoclonus or tremors can be observed during respiration in any structures of the oral cavity or pharynx including the tongue, soft palate, pharyngeal walls, or larynx.

Food Presentation Protocol: Lateral View

Measured liquid boluses. While seated and viewed in the lateral plane, the patient is given two to three swallows of each of the following materials: 1 ml, 3 ml, 5 ml, and 10 ml of liquid barium (as close to the consistency of water as possible). Each bolus is measured into a syringe. The 1- and 3-ml amounts are given on a spoon; 5- and 10-ml amounts are given in the syringe by placing the syringe between the patient's lips and gently releasing the material into the mouth (not squirting it posteriorly).

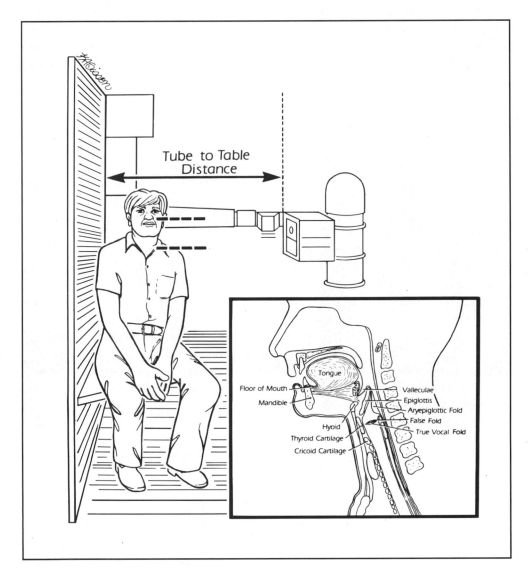

FIGURE 3.5.   The optimal positioning of a patient during the radiographic study, so that the entire oral cavity and pharynx are in view throughout the test.

Alternatively, the larger amounts of liquid can be measured into a syringe and given in an empty cup. In either procedure, the patient must be able to maintain lip closure to avoid losing material from the mouth. With each swallow, the patient is told to hold the material in his or her mouth until given the command to swallow. If the patient is unable to follow verbal directions, gestural communication can be used. The examiner may give the patient the material on a teaspoon and indicate that the patient is not to swallow by shaking a finger and/or the head negatively. If the patient is demented or completely unable to understand even gestural communication, the clinician may put the material in the patient's mouth and step back from the fluoroscopy machine quickly so that the equipment can be turned on and the swallow viewed. In this procedure, the oral stage may be missed, but the pharyngeal swallow will be captured. The clinician's hand should never be in the path of the X-ray beam in the process of placing the food in the patient's mouth.

Initially, the amount of liquid given per swallow is restricted in order to facilitate examination of the oral and pharyngeal structures and their movement, and to diminish the amount of aspiration that may occur. If a large liquid bolus (10 to 15 ml) were given initially, the radiopaque material would usually cover the structures and obliterate their movements. If a patient is at risk for aspiration, he or she may aspirate more on a larger bolus.

It is important that the X-ray tube remain focused on the oral cavity and pharynx after each swallow and throughout the entire procedure, as mentioned earlier. After each swallow a number of observations can be made that are critical to the identification and management of the patient's problem. For example, if the patient has residue in the pharynx after the swallow, the location of this residue before it is redistributed by gravity should be noted. Location of residue in the pharynx is an important symptom of various swallowing disorders, as discussed in Chapter 5. If the fluoroscopic tube drops to the esophagus after the pharyngeal swallow, the location of residue immediately after the swallow cannot be observed. Returning to view the pharynx after several seconds of examining the esophagus may produce erroneous observations of the location of residual food. Residue often moves by gravity after the swallow, particularly from the valleculae or pharyngeal walls into the pyriform sinuses. Accurate identification of pharyngeal swallowing disorders requires observation of the location of residual food immediately after the swallow.

It is equally important to note how the patient reacts to pharyngeal residue. Does he or she repeatedly dry swallow as a normal person would in response to feeling the residue in the pharynx? Or does the patient have no response to this residue because he or she has no awareness or realization that the material is left in the pharynx? Also, does any of this residue enter the airway after the swallow? Does the patient cough or clear the throat in response to this aspiration? Is this coughing productive in eliminating aspirated material? Aspiration after the swallow is a very common result of many swallowing disorders (Lazarus & Logemann, 1987; Logemann, 1985; Veis & Logemann, 1985).

It is equally important for the clinician to view the pharynx long enough after the swallow to identify whether aspiration of this residual material does occur. If the fluoroscopy tube follows the patient's swallow into the esophagus, important information on pharyngeal events that occur after the swallow in the handling of residual material will be lost. If the clinician decides to do a barium swallow and assess esophageal function (which is very important in the evaluation of swallowing disorders), this esophageal examination should be completed after the MBS procedure is completed.

In this way, no important information is lost during the procedure. Also, the MBS study will have carefully assessed the patient's risk of aspiration, so the esophageal study can be done more safely, or a decision can be made to postpone the esophageal study until the patient can swallow without significant aspiration.

If the clinician is concerned about aspiration of pharyngeal residue but no aspiration is observed after the swallow, the clinician can test the risk by viewing radiographically as patients turn their head to each side and lift their chin up and down. Head rotation to each side presses on each pyriform sinus. Lifting the chin up presses on the valleculae. If the residue in these pharyngeal recesses does not fall into the airway during these head movements, the risk is minimal that a patient will aspirate at a later time. The same procedure can be used with residue on pureed and solid foods.

Cup drinking. Cup drinking should be assessed in all patients who have not demonstrated any aspiration or significant residue on swallows of other volumes of liquid. Some patients who have an otherwise normal swallow exhibit dysfunction on cup drinking (Rasley et al., in press). During cup drinking, most individuals maintain airway closure and repeatedly take large (15- to 20-ml) quantities of material into their mouth and pharynx, swallowing each volume. Some patients will aspirate during the swallow because of reduced laryngeal closure during this task. It is important to examine these differences in physiology in any patient who has been successful in taking liquids in calibrated volumes, since most intake of liquids is done from a cup or a glass.

Saliva swallowing. In some patients, saliva swallowing should be evaluated. Though saliva is not radiopaque, the movement of oral and pharyngeal structures during a saliva swallow can be assessed. That is, movement of the tongue in the mouth and pharynx, laryngeal elevation, closure of the airway, and opening of the cricopharyngeal region (which will be narrow on a saliva swallow) can all be observed. The clinician can observe the saliva bolus after completing a traditional radiographic study, because a slight coating of barium will remain on the oropharyngeal structures, even in normal subjects. This barium will gradually mix with saliva so that observation of saliva swallows following swallows of traditional barium liquid and paste will often allow visualization of the saliva bolus itself during the swallow. Also, patients whose secretions pool in the pyriform sinuses can often be observed as a barium bolus mixes with the saliva before the pharyngeal swallow is triggered. The secretions can also often be observed in the laryngeal vestibule or overflowing from the pyriform sinus or sinuses into the laryngeal vestibule.

Paste and masticated boluses. When all liquid swallows are completed, two swallows of pudding mixed with barium should be given in ⅓-teaspoon (1-ml) amounts. Generally a mix of two parts pudding, one part pudding barium gives good contrast and good taste. A third swallow should be given if the patient's swallowing physiology differs on the first two swallows. The patient should be asked to hold the bolus and to begin the swallow on command. Again, gestural communication can be used.

When swallows of various volumes of thin liquid and two swallows of paste are completed, the clinician should give the patient one-fourth of a cookie (usually an easily chewed shortbread cookie, such as a Lorna Doone) with a small amount of the barium paste on the top for contrast. The patient is then told to chew the cookie, thereby mixing the barium with the cookie into a masticated bolus, and to begin the swallow whenever he or she is ready.

Eating. At times, observation of natural eating is important to understanding the patient's dysphagia. To observe eating, patients can be given a spoon and a bowl of pudding or other food mixed with barium and asked to eat the food as they normally would. In this way, the volume and speed the patients ordinarily use while eating can be observed in relation to their oral and pharyngeal swallowing physiology.

Food Presentation Protocol: Posterior-Anterior View

When the swallows of liquid, paste, and masticated materials have been completed in the lateral plane, the patient should be turned so that he or she can be viewed in the P-A plane. It is in this plane that the symmetry of the swallow can be assessed. In the P-A view, the two sides of the valleculae and the pyriform sinuses can be examined. Does material travel down the two sides equally? Is residue equal on the two sides? These questions can be answered in the P-A view. To keep radiation exposure to a minimum, only swallows of the food consistencies that were most difficult for the patient in the lateral view should be repeated in the P-A view.

While the patient is positioned for the examination in the P-A plane, it is also important to look at vocal fold function. The patient should be asked to tip his or her head backward to get the shadow of the mandible out of the way, as shown in Figure 3.6. Then, the patient should be asked to repeat "ah, ah, ah, ah" rapidly, so that the clinician can locate the vocal folds by identifying the area of soft tissue movement in the neck. The movement represents the adduction and abduction of the vocal folds. It is necessary to locate the vocal folds (soft tissue structures) during movement because on fluoroscopy the cervical spine lies behind the vocal folds, making identification of these soft tissues more difficult. With movement, however, the clinician can easily identify the location of the larynx and the true vocal folds.

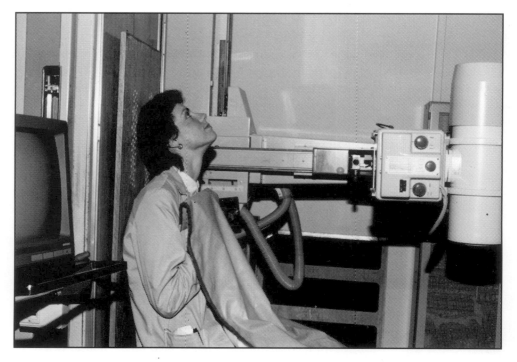

FIGURE 3.6. Positioning of the patient in the posterior-anterior plane, with the head elevated to allow visualization of the vocal folds.

The patient can then be asked to sustain phonation for several seconds, to pause for inhalation, and to sustain phonation for several more seconds. In this way, the clinician can examine vocal fold adduction and abduction and assess the symmetry of movement of the two sides of the larynx. Clearly, details of the vibratory cycle cannot be assessed in this way. However, the relative movement of the two sides of the larynx can be examined, and a unilateral adductor vocal fold paralysis can be identified.

Measuring Oropharyngeal Swallowing Parameters

It is often helpful to be able to measure the range of motion or temporal characteristics of selected aspects of the oropharyngeal swallow in order to document changes with recovery or degeneration or effects of treatment strategies, such as the Mendelsohn maneuver or the supersupraglottic swallow. In order to measure the movement of oropharyngeal structures during the swallow, the magnification introduced by the fluoroscopy equipment must be accounted for. This can be done by placing an object that serves as a "ruler" in the midline on the patient's neck or under the chin, as shown in Figure 3.7. Under the chin is usually best because it does not restrict laryngeal movement. Using a round object, such as a coin, will account for any slight changes in head position, since the maximum diameter of the coin will be the same, even if the patient moves slightly to the right or left.

Knowing the absolute diameter of the coin, the distance moved by any structure, such as the larynx, during swallow can be measured in absolute terms. So, for

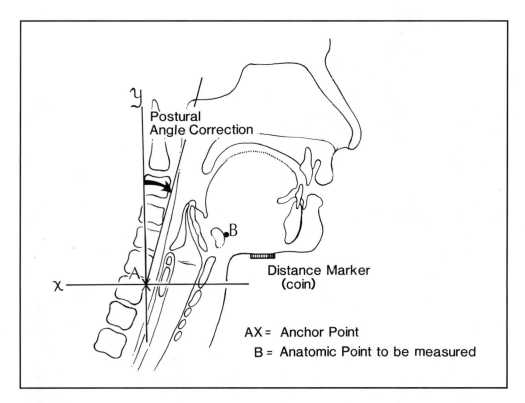

FIGURE 3.7. A lateral drawing of the oral cavity and pharynx illustrating the positioning of a coin or metal marker under the chin to enable measurement of real distance from the videofluoroscopic study. The patient's postural rotation from true vertical is also illustrated.

example, if the patient uses a Mendelsohn maneuver during the radiographic assessment, the clinician can measure the vertical movement of the larynx in millimeters during swallows in which the maneuver is used and those in which it is not used, in order to quantify the effect of the maneuver. Details of the procedure for measuring various aspects of the oropharyngeal swallow from radiographic studies are described in Chapter 6.

Report Writing

When the radiographic study is completed, a report of the study should be written. Details of the contents of the report are described in Chapter 8, and examples of reports for various types of patients are included in Chapter 9.

Patient-Family Counseling After the Videofluoroscopic Study

Videofluoroscopic assessment of swallowing is often the best tool to educate the family about the patient's swallowing physiology and techniques for improving the patient's function. Watching the radiographic study often makes clear to the family why the patient must assume a particular posture during eating, or why certain foods are dangerous to take by mouth. Whether the family is allowed to observe the radiographic study as it is being conducted, or whether the clinician chooses to provide a family education session using the videotaped record of the X-ray study after the MBS is completed, will depend on the clinician's awareness of the family's responsiveness and reaction to the patient's performance, as well as on time constraints. In general, families who have been counseled regarding the severity of their family member's swallowing impairment and the need for care in oral presentation of food prior to the X-ray study will be able to observe the X-ray study productively, as an aid to understanding their family member's disorders. However, some families, particularly familes of head-injured patients, have difficulty accepting the severity of the swallowing dysfunction. This is usually true in situations where the patient's swallow has not been previously assessed and the previous hospital or caregivers allowed the patient to take oral nutrition prior to any swallowing assessment. If the patient's performance is poor in the X-ray study and nonoral feeding is recommended, the family often does not accept this recommendation. They perceive the recommendation for nonoral feeding as removing a functional ability from the patient, who seems to them to be backsliding rather than progressing. Family members of the dysphagic patient need repeated counseling and support beginning prior to the evaluation period and continuing throughout treatment.

Radiation Safety

Throughout the radiographic study, it is important to keep radiation exposure to a minimum for the patient and the clinician. A patient in her childbearing years should be given a lead apron to wear throughout the procedure. The amount of radiation exposure the patient receives per minute of fluoroscopy will vary from machine to machine. The swallowing therapist should ask the radiation safety office at the hospital about the radiation generated by the particular fluoroscopic machine used at specific settings over a specified time, such as 1 min. A timer on the fluoroscopy machine will measure the duration of exposure for each patient, from which the patient's radiation exposure can be calculated.

The clinician should always wear a lead apron and a radiation badge, which is used to monitor total radiation exposure. If the clinician's hands are placed in the radiation field, he or she should wear lead-lined gloves. A lead collar to shield the thyroid from radiation exposure and leaded glasses to shield the eyes can be worn. If possible, the clinician should stand behind the lead shield of the control room during the study. Usually the clinician can do this by giving the patient the bolus to hold in his or her mouth until the clinician is positioned behind the lead shield. Then the patient can be given the command to swallow and the fluoroscopy machine turned on. If the clinician must stand next to the patient, as with infants and young children or many neurologically impaired or demented patients, portable lead shields can be positioned between the clinician and the fluoroscopy table, thus reducing the clinician's radiation exposure. The clinician should not hold a child's head or stabilize the jaw with an unprotected hand during the radiographic study.

NOTES

CHAPTER 4

Variations in the Modified
Barium Swallow Procedure

I n a number of instances the clinician will want to vary the MBS procedure just described because of the nature of a particular patient's medical status, behavioral characteristics, cognitive abilities, or swallowing disorders. Some of these variations are used from the beginning of the radiographic study, or the clinician may determine that these additional procedures are needed in the middle of the study or after the entire standard MBS examination has been completed, as described previously. Thus, some of the variations described in the following paragraphs are performed after the patient has completed the entire MBS study (14 or 16 swallows in the lateral and P-A planes), whereas others are introduced after one or two swallows.

Trial Therapy: Introduction of Management or Treatment Strategies to Improve the Patient's Swallow

A major purpose of the MBS is to identify treatment strategies that will improve the safety or efficiency of the patient's swallow. In this way, the patient may be allowed to eat under certain conditions rather than being committed to purely nonoral feeding or hydration. In general, treatment strategies should be introduced when a significant swallowing disorder is observed, that is, one that causes aspiration or a highly inefficient swallow with a great deal of oral or pharyngeal residue. The radiographic study should not always be terminated when a patient aspirates. Instead, a treatment strategy should be introduced that is selected based upon the nature of the patient's disorder. In general, treatment strategies are introduced in the radiographic study in the following order: (a) postural techniques, (b) increased sensory input, (c) treatment strategies, (d) volume changes, and (e) changes in diet or food consistency. This ordering of types of interventions reflects the ease with which a large variety of patients can use these techniques.

Postural techniques are introduced first because they can be applied to a large variety of patients, requiring no learning and minimal ability to follow directions (Horner et al., 1988; Kirchner, 1967; Logemann, 1986; Logemann, Kahrilas, Kobara, & Vakil, 1989; Shanahan, Logemann, Rademaker, Pauloski, & Kahrilas, in press; Welch, Logemann, Rademaker, & Kahrilas, 1993). Postural techniques have also been found to have a significant effect on the safety and efficiency of swallowing in many patients (Logemann, Kahrilas, Kobawa, & Valeil, 1989; Rasley et al., in press, Welch et al., 1993). If postural effects are inappropriate because of the nature of either the patient's swallowing problem or physical limitations, *changing sensory input* is another technique that requires relatively little cooperation or cognition on the patient's part. Increased sensory stimulation can be applied by the clinician without the need for the patient's active cooperation.

Swallowing therapy strategies such as voluntary control applied to the swallow (swallowing maneuvers), for example, the supraglottic swallow or the Mendelsohn maneuver, require cognition and ability to follow directions (Kahrilas et al., 1991; Logemann & Kahrilas, 1990). Therefore, these strategies are limited in application to patients who have good language and cognitive skills. These kinds of therapy techniques also often require increased energy on the part of the patient and their introduction can fatigue the patient more quickly. If a postural technique ameliorates the dysphagic symptoms (aspiration or residue), it is more efficient to use a postural change than to ask the patient to use a therapy strategy that will be fatiguing and may not be useful throughout a meal. However, some patients can only swallow safely and efficiently when using a swallowing maneuver or therapy technique (Logemann & Kahrilas, 1990). It is appropriate in many cases to attempt these techniques in X Ray, taking a few minutes to teach the patient the swallowing maneuver before turning on the fluoroscope and examining the revised swallowing physiology.

Once an effective set of interventions has been identified (postures, sensory stimulation, or maneuvers, or combinations of these), patients may be given _larger volumes_ of the same food, particularly liquids, to ensure that the strategies continue to work effectively on larger amounts. If the patient is unsuccessful in swallowing larger volumes using one or more of the techniques, the maximum volume that is tolerated well can be determined and recommended for oral intake. In some cases, the postural, sensory-stimulation, and treatment techniques alone or in combination work effectively throughout the volume range, and the patient can be permitted to take oral feeding when using the effective techniques with no volume restrictions. If this variety of strategies does not improve the patient's swallow on thin liquids, the clinician may decide to progress to _thicker foods,_ hypothesizing that the patient's disorder will not cause aspiration or significant residue on the thicker food consistency. If the patient's swallow is safe and/or efficient on thicker foods, oral feeding can be recommended on these thicker food consistencies, while eliminating oral intake of thick liquids or increasing the thickness of liquids by using a thickening product. By introducing treatment strategies in a systematic way during the radiographic study, the clinician can recommend specific constraints on oral intake rather than the complete elimination of oral nutrition or hydration.

The goal of the radiographic study is to maintain oral intake of foods that are safe and can be swallowed efficiently, even if it is under limited circumstances such as while using a particular postural technique or a particular swallowing maneuver. In Chapter 7 of this book, a number of examples are provided of protocols in which treatment techniques have been introduced. The protocols relate to particular swallowing disorders and are shown in Figures 7.1–7.4 and 7.6–7.8. These figures represent the sequence of presentation of various bolus types and treatment techniques. They are not meant to be prescriptions, but rather examples of the types of interventions introduced and the sequence of types of boluses given in concert with treatment strategies during the radiographic study.

It is very helpful to be able to assess the effectiveness of therapy procedures radiographically. Currently, there are only a few treatment or therapy techniques that can be performed quickly enough to be assessed during fluoroscopy. Many of the therapy techniques used in the management of oropharyngeal swallowing disorders, such as resistance and range-of-motion exercises or chewing exercises, are designed to improve neuromuscular control and require time to take effect (Logemann, 1983). Therefore, these techniques cannot be assessed while the patient is in Radiology. As new swallowing therapy techniques are devised, some additional treatment procedures may be examined fluoroscopically.

If the patient aspirates on a particular volume of liquid or other food, techniques to eliminate the aspiration should be introduced in the radiographic study. Usually, at least one swallow of liquid will be given to the patient according to the procedure outlined earlier before a decision is made to change this protocol. It is after this first swallow that the clinician may identify aspiration and its cause. Also, after the first liquid swallow, the clinician will probably have determined the patient's oral control in holding the bolus and initiating the swallow as well as his or her ability to protect the airway. In some cases, a second swallow may be given under the standard protocol. Therapy strategies may also be introduced if the patient's swallow is highly inefficient. As with aspiration, the etiology of the inefficiency will determine the nature of the strategies that are introduced. All of these physiologic considerations will determine whether or not the clinician decides to depart from the typical MBS procedure.

In the standard protocol, liquid volume is increased as long as no aspiration occurs. If aspiration occurs, the study should not be stopped. Instead, the clinician should examine the patient's swallowing physiology to determine the reason for the aspiration. The clinician should then introduce a change in the patient's posture designed to improve the swallow by eliminating the aspiration, unless there is no postural change that fits the patient's swallowing disorder. The particular posture selected will depend upon the physiologic reason for the aspiration. Table 4.1 presents swallowing postures and food consistencies that are often helpful for particular swallowing disorders. Another swallow of the same volume and bolus consistency as the one that was aspirated should be attempted while the patient uses the posture to determine whether or not the posture has, in fact, improved the swallow. If the aspiration has been eliminated, the patient can proceed through the rest of the study, including larger volumes of liquid while using the same postural change. If the postural change is not effective on a particular volume, a swallowing maneuver may be introduced alone or in combination with a postural change.

TABLE 4.1   Postures and Food Consistencies Most Often Helpful to Patients with Particular Swallowing Disorders

SWALLOWING DISORDER	POSTURE	FOOD CONSISTENCY
Tongue dysfunction	Chin up	Thickened liquids
Delayed pharyngeal swallow	Chin down	Thickened liquids, purees
Reduced posterior motion of tongue base	Chin down	Liquids and thickened liquids
Unilateral pharyngeal paresis	Head rotated to damaged side	Liquids, thinner foods
Unilateral tongue and pharyngeal weakness, same side	Lean toward stronger, unaffected side	Liquids and thickened liquids
Bilateral pharyngeal weakness	Lie on side or back	Liquids, thinner foods
Reduced laryngeal closure	Chin down, head rotated to damaged side	Purees
Reduced laryngeal elevation	Chin down, Lie on side or back	Purees
Cricopharyngeal dysfunction, reduced anterior laryngeal movement	Head rotated to either side	Liquids

Postural Variations

There are a number of postural variations that may change pharyngeal dimensions (Logemann, Kahrilas, Kobara, & Vakil, 1989, Welch et al., 1993) or the gravitational flow of food through the oral cavity and pharynx and that may, therefore, reduce the patient's aspiration and increase the amount of material entering the esophagus. Postural variations do not change the patient's disordered swallowing physiology. Rather, they are compensatory techniques that are, it is hoped, used as temporary measures to improve food intake while the patient recovers spontaneously or undergoes swallowing therapy directed at improving the underlying swallowing physiology. If the swallowing therapist feels that a postural change will improve the patient's speed of oral intake or reduce the amount of aspiration, the patient's posture should be changed and additional swallows examined while the patient uses the posture during the radiographic study. This will facilitate the careful assessment of the effects of each posture and enable the swallowing therapist to demonstrate these effects to the patient's attending physicians, other health care professionals, and family members. Not all postures described here should be tried with each patient. The selection of a particular posture for a particular patient should not be haphazard; instead, the clinician should choose the posture that is most appropriate for the patient's specific swallowing problems. This choice is based upon the physiologic or anatomic swallowing disorders observed during the initial swallows.

Tilting the head forward, chin down. Tilting the patient's head forward, chin down, pushes the anterior wall of the pharynx posteriorly, significantly narrowing the airway entrance and pushing the tongue base and the epiglottis significantly farther backward toward the posterior pharyngeal wall (Welch et al., 1993). In some patients, the chin-down posture results in a widened vallecular space as the tongue falls forward and the epiglottis falls somewhat backward. These changes are illustrated in Figure 4.1. Some clinicians recommend this posture for *all* patients with dysphagia, but following this type of dictum can only lead some patients to increased difficulty in swallowing. The key to the successful use of posture to improve swallowing is to select the particular posture to match the individual patient's physiology and anatomy. This requires knowledge of the individual patient's anatomic and physiologic status.

The head-down (chin-down) posture is often helpful for the patient with a delayed pharyngeal swallow (or reflex), since it narrows the airway entrance and increases the vallecular space, thereby increasing the probability that the material swallowed will sit in the valleculae prior to the triggering of the pharyngeal swallow, decreasing the risk of aspiration. This posture is also often helpful for patients with poor laryngeal closure during the swallow. With the head tilted down, the epiglottis tends to divert material away from the top of the airway so that the chance of aspiration is reduced. The chin-down posture can also be helpful in patients with reduced tongue-base retraction, since it pushes the tongue base closer to the pharyngeal wall. This posture is not appropriate for patients with reduced pharyngeal contraction or reduced tongue control.

The chin-down posture is less apt to be helpful in eliminating aspiration in patients with a delayed pharyngeal swallow if the bolus drops to the pyriform sinuses during the pharyngeal delay (Shanahan et al., in press). The chin-down posture has no documented effect on the dimensions of the pyriform sinuses. When the pharyngeal swallow is triggered, the larynx and pharynx immediately elevate, thus shortening the pyriform sinus. If the bolus has collected in the pyriform sinus during the delay in the

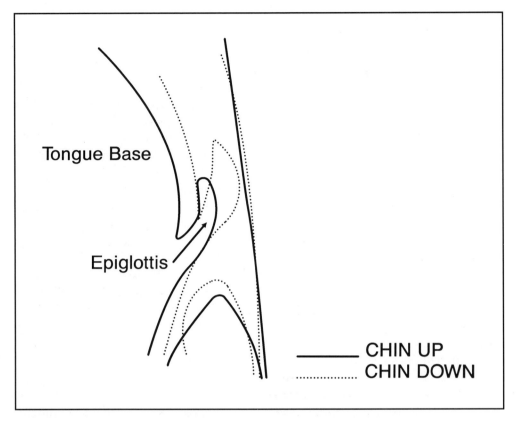

FIGURE 4.1.   A lateral drawing of the oral cavity and pharynx illustrating the changes in pharyngeal dimensions created with the chin-down position.

pharyngeal swallow, the food will be dumped into the airway as the pyriform sinus elevates and shortens with the pharynx (Shanahan et al., in press). Since some patients in this situation do benefit from the chin-down posture, the effects of the posture should still be evaluated as a part of the radiographic study.

Tilting the head backward.   Tilting the head backward facilitates gravitational drainage of food out of the oral cavity and thus improves the speed of oral transit time (OTT) in those patients with poor tongue control or with part of the tongue surgically removed (Logemann, 1983). The chin-down posture can be combined with the head-back posture in patients who tend to lose control of food when it is placed in their mouth. In this case, patients are asked to place food in the mouth while the head is down and are then instructed to throw the head backward when they are ready to begin the swallow. This prevents the premature loss of food from the oral cavity into the pharynx prior to the initiation of the swallow. If the clinician is concerned that patients will aspirate food before the pharyngeal swallow can be triggered when their head is tilted backward, the patients can be taught to close their airway voluntarily (the supraglottic swallow) before tossing their head back. In this way, the airway is closed before the start of the swallow and food falling into the pharynx cannot be aspirated.

Rotating the head to the damaged side.   Rotating the head to one side closes the pyriform sinus on that side (Kirchner, 1967; Logemann, Kahrilas, Kobara, & Vakil, 1989). Thus, patients with unilateral pharyngeal weakness or paralysis can benefit from turning their head to the paralyzed side and directing food down the opposite or stronger side (see Figure 4.2). In all cases, the patient's head should be turned toward the damaged side. Turning the head also places external pressure on the vocal fold on the side toward which the patient turns. This external pressure on the damaged vocal cord moves it toward the midline, thus improving airway closure. Patients with reduced airway closure because of a unilateral laryngeal weakness or paralysis, or patients who have had part of their larynx removed unilaterally (e.g., hemilaryngectomy), may benefit from turning the head toward the damaged side.

Head rotation combined with chin down.   Generally, the best airway closure is accomplished by combining head rotation to the impaired side with a chin-down posture. Head rotation pushes the damaged vocal fold closer to the midline and directs the bolus away from the damaged side of the larynx, while the chin-down posture narrows the airway entrance dimension. Some patients benefit from the combined postures and their aspiration is eliminated, although they do not benefit from either posture used separately.

Tilting the head to the stronger side.   Tilting the head toward the stronger side tends to direct material down that side, both in the oral cavity and in the pharynx. This is an appropriate posture for patients with both unilateral tongue dysfunction *and* unilateral pharyngeal disorders on the *same side.* The patient should always tilt toward his or her better side and should have the head tilted when food is placed in the mouth. Otherwise, food will fall to the damaged side before the patient can move his or her head into position.

Lying on the 'side or back.   Patients who aspirate after the swallow because of residue in the pharynx are aspirating because gravity drops the residual food into the airway when they inhale after the swallow. Some of these patients may benefit from lying on one side or on their back during swallowing to prevent this aspiration after the swallow. Usually these are patients with reduced pharyngeal contraction (peristal-

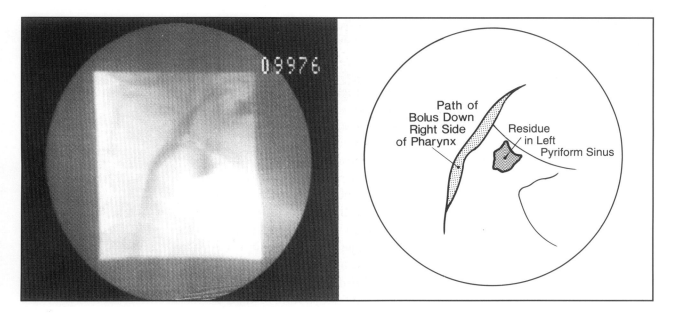

FIGURE 4.2.   A lateral radiographic view of a patient with the head rotated to the left during swallow. The bolus being swallowed can be seen flowing down one side of the pharynx, while residual food remains in the opposite pyriform sinus. Head rotation results in closure of one side of the pharynx with food directed down the opposite side.

sis) or reduced laryngeal elevation who have residue in the valleculae and/or pyriform sinuses but whose residue does not increase with successive swallows. If the pharyngeal residue increases with successive swallows, it will overflow into the airway despite any postural changes. Patients who benefit from lying down are those who normally aspirate after the swallow because of chronic residue after the swallow. That is, each successive swallow pushes the residue from the previous swallow into the esophagus so that there is always a constant amount of food remaining in the pharynx after the swallow. These patients chronically aspirate because of the effect of gravity on this residue. When the patients are laid on one side or on their back, the direction of gravity is changed, holding the bolus on the pharyngeal walls so that no aspiration occurs. They can then begin eating in this posture and can be reassessed monthly for any recovery of function. Usually, the etiology of the reduced pharyngeal contraction or reduced laryngeal elevation in these patients is either stroke, head trauma, or a surgical procedure for head-and-neck cancer, so that some recovery is anticipated (Lazarus & Logemann, 1987; Logemann, 1985; Veis & Logemann, 1985). It is unlikely that this supine or side-lying posture would be helpful for any length of time in a patient with degenerative neurologic disease, such as amyotrophic lateral sclerosis.

Some of the older literature on management of dysphagic patients indicates that patients should never lie down to swallow. This type of strict protocol assumes that every dysphagic patient has similar swallowing physiology. This is clearly not the case. Posture should be matched to the patient's oropharyngeal anatomy and swallowing physiology. Many patients who are in the process of recovery after neurologic or structural damage, and whose last remaining swallowing disorder is reduced pharyngeal contraction or reduced laryngeal elevation, may be positioned in a side-lying or supine position to facilitate eating. The clinician should be sure, however, that the patient has no esophageal or gastric disorder that may cause reflux and reentry of material into the pharynx. If the patient suffers from reflux, the problem may worsen when he or she is in the supine or side-lying position, and this may put the patient at increased risk of aspiration of refluxed material.

Summary of postural changes. Using the videofluorographic procedure to assess the effects of posture on the movement of food and on the presence of aspiration in a particular patient can be important in returning the patient to oral feeding more quickly and in educating other health professionals and the family regarding the effect of posture on the patient's swallowing ability. It must be stressed that changing posture does not modify the patient's swallowing physiology; instead, it changes oropharyngeal dimensions and the pathway of food flow and thus often changes the amount of food that enters the esophagus as opposed to the airway.

Postural changes are purely compensatory (i.e., they do not change the patient's physiologic capability or neuromuscular control). Rather, they are used as temporary measures to facilitate safe and more efficient eating while the patient undergoes therapy to improve neuromuscular function and recovers so that the postural options are no longer needed. When postural options are used, the patient's swallowing physiology should be reassessed regularly using videofluorography, usually at 4- to 6-week intervals, to evaluate recovery and determine when the postures are no longer needed. During the reevaluation, the patient should be examined initially in the usual upright eating position. This enables assessment of the patient's deglutition without the postural intervention. If the patient's swallowing physiology has recovered, the examination can proceed to increased liquid volumes and viscosities to assure that physiology is adequate across bolus types. If the patient aspirates on a particular volume or viscosity, the postural technique can be reintroduced.

In general, postural changes are relatively easy for a patient to implement and do not increase the patient's fatigue. This makes them applicable to patients who fatigue easily, such as those with motor neuron disease, as well as to a wide range of other types of patients.

Increasing Sensory Input

Another set of strategies that can be introduced in the radiographic study to improve the patient's swallowing physiology is increased oral sensory stimulation prior to the swallow. Generally, this set of strategies is appropriate for a patient with reduced recognition of food in the mouth or very slowed oral transit because of an apraxic component. This increased sensory stimulation may take a number of forms including (a) increasing the downward pressure of the spoon against the tongue as the bolus is delivered into the mouth; (b) introducing a bolus with increased sensory characteristics, such as a cold bolus or a textured bolus (e.g., rice pudding) or a bolus with a strong flavor; (c) providing a bolus requiring chewing so that the mastication provides preliminary oral stimulation; (d) thermal-tactile stimulation to the anterior faucial arches prior to the swallow; and (e) providing a larger-volume bolus. Some patients respond to one or more of these techniques by producing a more normal swallow, particularly in the onset and speed of the oral stage and in the triggering of the pharyngeal swallow. For some patients, the motor act of swallowing appears to begin with the arm-and-hand action of the feeding act itself. These patients do best when they are given the spoon containing the desired bolus and are allowed to place the food in the mouth themselves. These patients may show no oral tongue motion or other response when food is placed in the mouth for them, but when they place food in their own mouth, there is normal onset of tongue movement and speed of the oral stage of swallowing. Like postural changes, techniques to increase sensory input do not fatigue the patient and are relatively easy to implement in a wide variety of patients.

Thermal-tactile stimulation is designed to improve the speed of triggering of the pharyngeal swallow in patients who have been identified from assessment of previous swallows as having a delay in triggering the pharyngeal swallow (Lazzara, Lazarus, & Logemann, 1986). Thermal-tactile stimulation should only be done when a delay in triggering the pharyngeal swallow has been defined radiographically on at least *two* consecutive swallows. Some neurologically impaired patients, such as patients with cerebrovascular accidents, exhibit a "warm-up" period when eating, so that triggering of the pharyngeal swallow may be most delayed on the first swallow and may improve somewhat on the second swallow. Thus, the second swallow may be more representative of the patient's usual functional pattern than the first swallow.

To perform thermal-tactile stimulation and assess the effects radiographically, the patient is asked to open his or her mouth while the clinician places a cold, size-00 laryngeal mirror at the base of the anterior faucial arch (Figure 4.3). Complete contact of the back side of the laryngeal mirror to the faucial arch is maintained while rubbing the mirror up and down vertically five times. The mirror is then removed and placed in ice again for several seconds. The stimulation is repeated on the opposite side of the oral cavity, if both sides are equally sensitive. In the case of oral surgical patients, the contact is always made on the unoperated side of the oral cavity. If the patient has a bite reflex and may bite on the mirror, injury to the patient can be prevented by coating the mirror and handle with Teflon so that the metal back side of the mirror used for the stimulation is left uncoated (Helfrich-Miller, personal communication, 1984).

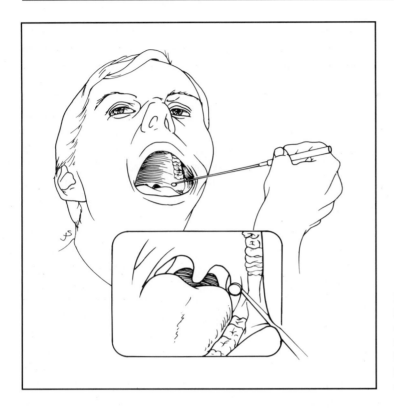

FIGURE 4.3. A front view of the oral cavity illustrating the thermal-tactile stimulation technique applied to the anterior faucial arches.

Upon completion of the stimulation, the patient is immediately given a small amount of iced liquid barium and told to swallow it. The swallow following thermal-tactile stimulation is then assessed radiographically and compared to similar swallows completed without such stimulation. Results of a study by Lazzara et al. (1986) indicate that 95% of the patients identified radiographically as having a delay in triggering of the pharyngeal swallow will improve in speed after thermal-tactile stimulation. This 1986 study does not address the role of thermal-tactile stimulation in the recovery of functional swallowing but documents the immediate effects of the procedure.

The clinician can then use the videotaped example of the immediate effects of thermal-tactile stimulation in education of the patient's family, physician, and other health care professionals regarding the rationale for the procedure. It is important to note that thermal-tactile stimulation does not trigger the pharyngeal swallow at the time of the stimulation. Rather, the purpose of the stimulation is to *heighten the sensitivity* for the swallow in the central nervous system and to alert the central nervous system so that when the patient voluntarily attempts to swallow, he or she will trigger a pharyngeal swallow more rapidly (Logemann, 1983).

Voluntary Maneuvers to Protect the Airway

At various times, normal subjects and dysphagic patients use a variety of voluntary maneuvers to protect the airway before and during the swallow. In normal subjects, anterior tilting of the arytenoid cartilage to contact the base of the epiglottis can often be observed in anticipation of swallows of a large volume (10 ml or larger, as in cup drinking). For example, when a normal subject brings a cup of liquid to the lips, it is common to see the arytenoid tilt toward the base of the epiglottis, closing the airway entrance, as liquid is taken into the mouth, before the oral or pharyngeal swallow is initiated. This behavior can also be observed in some dysphagic patients.

A chin-down posture is sometimes used spontaneously by patients in an attempt to protect the airway during swallow. Another postural technique sometimes used is chin retraction, in which the chin is pulled backward, pushing the tongue base closer to the pharyngeal wall and again narrowing the laryngeal inlet. Any one of these maneuvers observed during a radiographic study may be interpreted as a compensatory strategy used by the patient in an attempt to protect the airway.

Supraglottic swallow. The goal of the supraglottic swallow is to close the vocal folds before and during the swallow, thus protecting the trachea from aspiration (Logemann, 1983), as illustrated in Figure 4.4. The supraglottic swallow or the voluntary airway closure technique can be attempted with a patient for the first time during the fluoroscopy session. The patient must be alert, relatively relaxed, and able to follow simple directions without becoming upset or confused. The clinician can direct the patient through the procedure step by step during the radiographic study. To do this, the patient is given material to swallow and is told to keep it in his or her mouth while directions are given. The directions should be as follows:

1. Take a deep breath and hold your breath.

2. Keep holding your breath and lightly cover your tracheostomy tube (if a tracheostomy is present).

3. Keep holding your breath while you swallow.

4. Immediately after the swallow, cough.

These steps should be practiced with the patient on saliva swallows prior to giving him or her the actual food to swallow. However, the patient cannot take a great deal of time to practice while in Radiology. If he or she is able to follow the directions correctly several times without food, the procedure may be tried under fluoroscopy with some expectation of success. At all times, the clinician should continue to provide verbal directions for each step.

If the patient becomes confused or cannot follow directions easily, this technique should not be tried initially during the MBS. Instead, the patient should be returned to his or her room and the clinician should work with the patient until the technique has been learned. When the supraglottic procedure has been mastered, the patient can be rescheduled for another fluorographic study and the success of this technique in improving airway closure can be assessed. If the patient has a large gap in glottic closure, as may be seen following extended partial laryngectomy or in bilateral adductor paralysis, the supraglottic swallow procedure alone will not be sufficient to achieve airway protection. The patient will also need adduction exercises, which must be practiced for a week or more before improvement in vocal cord adduction can be expected (Logemann, 1983).

In some patients, the direction "Take a deep breath and hold your breath" does not result in vocal fold closure. Instead, some patients hold their breath by stopping chest wall movement. These patients appear to be performing the supraglottic swallow procedure correctly, but fluorographic examination of the swallow reveals an open airway. For these patients, a change in instructions is needed. The clinician can instruct

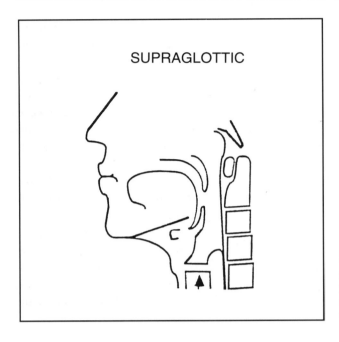

SUPRAGLOTTIC

FIGURE 4.4.   A lateral diagram of the oral cavity and pharynx illustrating the focus of the supraglottic swallow on closure of the true vocal folds.

the patient: "Inhale and then exhale slightly; hold your breath and swallow while holding your breath." Since the vocal folds move toward each other slightly during exhalation, holding the breath on exhalation may result in vocal fold closure. Alternatively, the clinician may tell the patient, "Inhale and then say 'Ah'; stop voicing and hold your breath." Usually, one of these techniques will elicit vocal fold closure on the breath hold.

Extended supraglottic swallow—the "dump and swallow" technique.   Some patients with severe reductions in tongue mobility or severely reduced tongue bulk because of surgical procedures for oral cancer essentially have little or no oral transit. They need to take a sufficient volume of liquid to drop the bolus by gravity from the mouth to the pharynx with chin elevation (extension). During the radiographic study, these patients should be taught the extended supraglottic swallow or "dump and swallow" technique. First, these patients should be given very small amounts (1 ml or 3 ml) of liquid on a spoon. These small-volume swallows should be observed as the patient tosses his or her head back and dumps the liquid into the pharynx to determine whether (a) the pharyngeal swallow is triggered on time and (b) airway closure is sufficient to protect the airway. If both airway closure and triggering of the pharyngeal swallow are normal, the patient can be given 5 to 10 ml of liquid in a cup and taught the following sequence:

1. Hold your breath tightly.

2. Put the entire 5 to 10 ml of liquid in your mouth.

3. Continue to hold your breath and toss your head back, thus dumping the liquid into the pharynx as a whole.

4. Swallow two to three times or as many times as needed to clear the majority of the liquid *while continuing to hold your breath.*

5. Cough to clear any residue from the pharynx.

This process is much like a normal swallow when consecutive swallows of liquid are taken from a cup. Normal swallowers usually hold their breath throughout all of the consecutive swallows.

As the patient's confidence and efficiency with the procedure increase, up to 30 ml may be taken at one time, using five to six repeated swallows while holding the airway closed. Figure 4.5 illustrates this technique. At the end of the sequence of swallows, the patient should cough to clear any residual food from the pharynx. This technique enables the patient with severe lingual impairment to take a significant amount of calories in a short period of time.

Supersupraglottic swallow.   The supersupraglottic swallow is designed to close the entrance to the airway voluntarily by tilting the arytenoid cartilage anteriorly to the base of the epiglottis before and during the swallow, as illustrated in Figure 4.6. This is the normal mechanism for closure of the entrance to the airway; it is facilitated during normal swallowing by the elevation of the larynx. Laryngeal elevation brings the arytenoid cartilage closer to the posterior surface of the epiglottis, so that the arytenoid does not have to move as far anteriorly. The effort involved in the supersupraglottic swallow increases the anterior tilt of the arytenoid to close the entrance to the airway early, both before and during the swallow. The patient is given the following

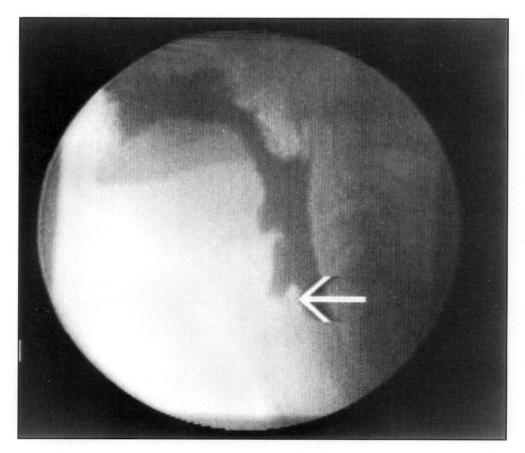

FIGURE 4.5.   A lateral videoprint of the "dump and swallow" technique with a liquid bolus of approximately 20 ml stretching from the lips anteriorly to the pyriform sinuses inferiorly. The arrow indicates closure of the airway. The patient will now swallow repeatedly five or six times to clear this bolus. The swallows will be followed by a final cough to clear any residue from the airway entrance.

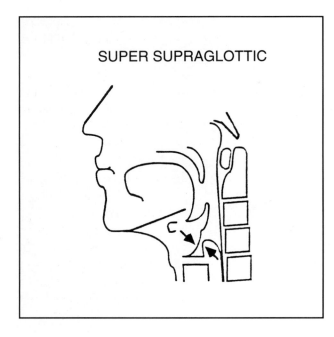

FIGURE 4.6.   A lateral diagram of the oral cavity and pharynx showing the focus of the supersupraglottic swallow on closure of the entrance to the airway between the arytenoid cartilage and the base of epiglottis.

instructions: "Inhale and hold your breath very tightly, bearing down. Keep holding your breath and bearing down as you swallow."

Bearing down helps to tilt the arytenoid forward and close the entrance to the airway. This strategy is used in patients with reduced closure of the airway entrance, particularly those who have undergone a supraglottic laryngectomy. During supraglottic laryngectomy, the epiglottis is removed and the laryngeal entrance consists of the tongue base and arytenoid cartilage. These differences in anatomy of the airway entrance or vestibule are illustrated in Figure 4.7. In the case of the supraglottic laryngectomy, the arytenoid cartilage tilts forward to contact the tongue base, rather than the base of the epiglottis. In the supraglottic laryngectomy, the supersupraglottic swallow improves tongue-base retraction as well as the anterior tilt of the arytenoid. The supersupraglottic swallow can also be used as an exercise to improve tongue-base retraction in patients with normal anatomy.

Voluntary Maneuvers to Improve Clearance of the Bolus

Patients with reduced tongue movement may spontaneously *toss the head back* to use gravity to assist in clearing food from the oral cavity. These same patients often gravitate to thinner food consistencies, which require less lingual pressure to clear from the oral cavity and move more easily by gravity (Dantas et al., 1989; Dantas et al., 1990).

Patients with residual food left in the pharynx after the swallow may exhibit several voluntary behaviors in an attempt to reduce the residue. A *chin-down posture* during swallowing may be used to push the tongue base posteriorly, narrowing the distance between the tongue base and the pharyngeal wall and thus reducing the distance the tongue base needs to move. The chin-down posture may eliminate residue in the valleculae.

Another strategy for managing residue in the pharynx after the swallow is *spontaneous dry swallowing*. If the patient is aware of pharyngeal residue after the first swallow of a bolus, he or she will typically swallow again immediately to clear this

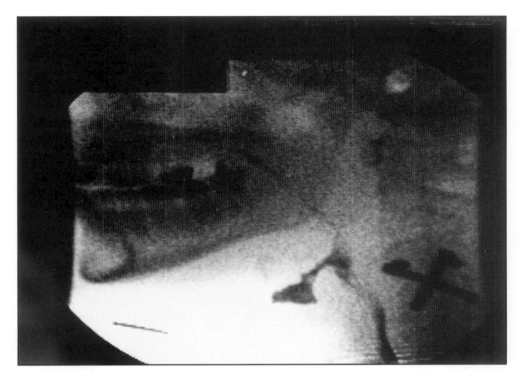

FIGURE 4.7. A lateral videoprint illustrating the anatomic changes after supraglottic laryngectomy, with the tongue base ending at the vocal folds.

residue. Some patients will use three to five spontaneous dry swallows to clear residue. Use of the spontaneous dry swallow indicates good pharyngeal sensation. If a patient is not aware of food remaining in the pharynx, and therefore does not spontaneously dry swallow, he or she may be taught to voluntarily dry swallow after each food swallow to clear the residue. It may be more productive to have the patient alternate liquids and solids as described below, since a dry swallow is more work for no additional calories.

Washing food through the pharynx. Washing food through the pharynx may be helpful to patients who have excessive residue in the pharynx after the swallow and do not automatically dry swallow or in whom the dry-swallow technique may not be successful in clearing the remaining material from the pharynx. Also, a liquid wash provides increased hydration. In these cases, it is often helpful to give the patient water or liquid barium during videofluoroscopy to assess the effect of liquid in washing food through the pharynx. In this case, the patient is given half a cup of water or other liquid and told to take a small sip and hold it in the mouth until asked to swallow. If the patient cannot be trusted to take only a small amount of water or other liquid, the clinician may present ⅓ to ½ teaspoon of water on a spoon. This can be repeated as many times as desired until the residue is cleared from the pharynx.

Effortful swallow. The effortful swallow is a technique designed to improve tongue-base movement posteriorly and thus improve clearance of the bolus from the valleculae, as illustrated in Figure 4.8. In this voluntary maneuver, the patient is given the following instructions: "As you swallow, push and squeeze with all of the muscles of your mouth and throat. Try to swallow 'hard,' squeezing hard all the way through the

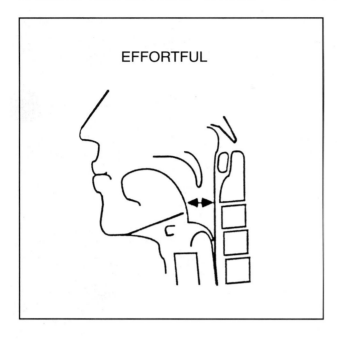

EFFORTFUL

FIGURE 4.8.   A lateral drawing of the oral cavity and pharynx illustrating the focus of the effortful swallow on decreasing the distance between the tongue base and posterior pharyngeal wall during the pharyngeal stage of swallow.

swallow." As the patient uses this maneuver, there should be improved clearance of the bolus from the valleculae and improved posterior tongue-base movement.

Mendelsohn maneuver.   The Mendelsohn maneuver uses information on the biomechanics of cricopharyngeal opening to improve laryngeal elevation and cricopharyngeal opening during the swallow (Kahrilas et al., 1991; Logemann & Kahrilas, 1990). The Mendelsohn maneuver is designed to improve laryngeal elevation and the duration and width of cricopharyngeal opening during the swallow, as illustrated in Figure 4.9. To teach the patient the Mendelsohn maneuver, the clinician asks the patient to concentrate on the feeling in his or her neck during a swallow and to determine whether he or she can feel the larynx (Adam's apple or voice box) lifting during the swallow and lowering after the swallow. Most patients who need the Mendelsohn maneuver have restricted laryngeal elevation but can still perceive that the larynx moves upward somewhat as they attempt to swallow. When patients have tried several saliva swallows and indicate that they can feel their voice box lifting and coming back down during the swallow, they are given the following instructions: "Swallow normally and feel with your muscles how the voice box lifts when you swallow. As you swallow and the voice box lifts to the top of your neck, *don't let it come back down* for several seconds. Hold it up with your muscles. Don't lift your voice box early. Just swallow normally and as your voice box lifts and gets to the top of your throat, hold it up with your muscles and don't let it drop for several seconds."

Studies of normal subjects performing this maneuver indicate that they follow the directions exactly, not preelevating the larynx, but holding it up for several seconds as it reaches its elevated position (Kahrilas et al., 1991). When the larynx is held in an elevated position during the swallow, the duration of cricopharyngeal opening is prolonged. In patients with reduced laryngeal elevation and/or reduced cricopharyngeal opening, this maneuver will facilitate increased laryngeal lifting and increased duration and width of cricopharyngeal opening. Most patients use this maneuver for only a few months as their swallow recovers. They do not need to use it permanently.

However, we have had several patients who had to use the maneuver permanently in order to eat both safely and efficiently (Logemann & Kahrilas, 1990).

Summary

At this time, the foregoing techniques are the only therapeutic procedures that are simple enough for the patient to learn quickly and easily in Radiology. The clinician should avoid attempting to teach the patient techniques in Radiology that are time-consuming to learn. If more than 5 to 10 min. of teaching time are required, the clinician should plan to see the patient at a later time at the bedside to accomplish the necessary teaching and should reschedule the patient for a second or *continued* MBS study at a later date, when sufficient teaching and learning has taken place.

When reevaluating a patient who is using a postural or therapy technique during eating, it is best to begin the study by asking the patient *not* to use the treatment technique. In this way, the swallowing therapist can observe the patient's baseline swallow and determine if recovery has taken place. The patient may no longer need the postural or therapy technique in order to eat safely and efficiently. It is important to note that even if patients are not voluntarily using any swallowing maneuvers, remnants of these procedures may have been habituated and incorporated into their baseline swallowing pattern.

Special Populations

There are many types of dysphagic patients who require specific modifications in the videofluorographic study of oropharyngeal swallowing in order to complete the study successfully and in order for the clinician to collect accurate information regarding their oropharyngeal swallowing physiology. Among these patients are infants, young children, head-injured individuals, adults or children with mental retardation or developmental delay, individuals with cerebral palsy and other movement disorders,

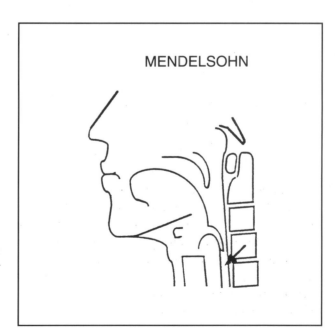

FIGURE 4.9. A lateral drawing of the oral cavity and pharynx illustrating the focus of the Mendelsohn maneuver on the opening of the upper esophageal sphincter during the pharyngeal stage of swallow.

ventilator-dependent patients, spinal-cord-injured patients who are immobilized with various types of bracing, patients with oral apraxia, and patients whose alertness is reduced. The procedural considerations that are most important for effective evaluation of these patients are discussed below. In general, all of these types of patients take more time in the radiographic suite than does the typical stroke patient or postoperative head-and-neck surgical patient. Patience with these individuals and anticipation of some of their special needs will reward the examiner with a videofluorographic swallowing study that accurately reflects the individual's typical oropharyngeal swallowing physiology.

Spinal-Cord-Injured Patients with Bracing

Spinal-cord-injured patients are often stabilized and may not be able to be elevated fully to a complete vertical position, or they may be elevated only when some type of neck or chin brace is present. If the patient cannot be elevated, the radiographic study should be completed in the patient's usual position, that is, the position in which he or she is usually fed. This may be at 30° or 60° above horizontal. If spinal-cord-injured patients are braced, they often comment that they feel as if the bracing makes their swallowing more difficult. A recent study that examined the effects of a somi brace on normal swallowing physiology revealed no change in any oral or pharyngeal swallowing measures except duration of airway closure, which was significantly longer with than without bracing (Bisch, Logemann, Rademaker, & Quigley, 1992). This difference may result from subjects' compensating for the discomfort of the brace. All of the normal subjects, like most spinal-cord-injured patients, commented that it felt more uncomfortable to swallow with the brace in place.

With head-and-neck bracing in place, certain parts of the oral cavity or pharynx may be shadowed or covered by the brace, as shown in Figure 4.10. If this is the case, the patient's wheelchair or cart may need to be angled slightly to reveal these structures. Usually, angling the chair or cart 15° to 30° from straight lateral will sufficiently move the shadow of the bracing away from critical anatomic elements of the pharynx. The radiographic view is not strictly lateral with the cart or wheelchair at an angle, but in these patients, the bracing cannot be removed. And, in most cases, it is not appropriate to delay the radiographic study until the bracing is removed, since many of these patients will wear bracing for a number of months, during which time they might potentially be full or partial oral feeders if their swallow is found to be functional. If swallowing abnormalities are seen, the patients can receive swallowing therapy to restore their swallowing physiology to a functional status.

Tracheotomized Patients

Before beginning the radiographic study, the clinician should examine the tracheostomy tube of tracheotomized patients to determine the presence of a cuff and its status (inflated or deflated), the size of the tracheostomy tube, and the presence of a fenestration. The clinician should also review the patient's chart to determine the length of time the tracheostomy has been in place. If the tracheostomy tube has been in place more than 6 months, scar tissue may have formed that can restrict laryngeal elevation. Tracheostomy tubes in place for a shorter time may have no effect on laryngeal elevation if the cuff is deflated. If it is medically feasible, the tracheostomy cuff should be deflated during the radiographic study, since an inflated cuff can reduce laryngeal elevation by creating friction against the tracheal wall. However, the tra-

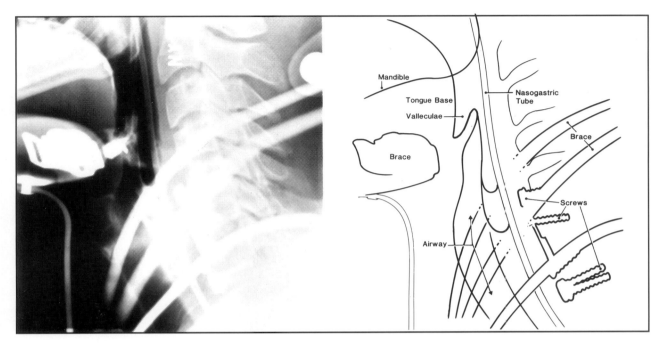

FIGURE 4.10. A lateral radiographic view of the pharynx in a patient who has undergone cervical spinal fusion, showing both bracing and the hardware involved in fusion. The patient has a nasogastric tube in place.

cheostomy cuff should not be deflated until medical clearance is given. If the cuff is inflated during the radiographic study, the clinician should note this in the report.

The patient with a tracheostomy tube should be taught to lightly cover the external end of the tube with a gauze pad during the moment of the swallow and for several seconds after the swallow. In this way, increased airflow is directed through the larynx, which stimulates subglottic sensory receptors before the swallow and may improve vocal fold closure. Most swallows occur during the exhalatory phase of the respiratory cycle, with exhalation temporarily stopped by the swallow (Martin, 1991). Exhalation usually resumes after the swallow. Thus, if the patient's tracheostomy is occluded during and immediately after the swallow, the exhalatory airflow after the swallow potentially contributes to clearance of residual food away from the top of the airway, lessening the chance of aspiration after the swallow. It is also thought that covering the tracheostomy tube helps to restore more normal subglottic pressures during swallowing and thus also helps to improve closure of the vocal folds during deglutition. The clinician may want to evaluate the tracheotomized patient's swallow with the tracheotomy tube covered and uncovered to assess the difference in safety and efficiency. Many patients aspirate with the tube uncovered and do not aspirate with it covered.

Ventilator-Dependent Patients

Ventilator-dependent patients can be seen for a videofluoroscopic evaluation of swallowing either on a portable ventilator or by receiving ventilation by Ambu bag from a respiratory therapist or nurse who accompanies the patient to radiology. Usually, these patients are seen on a cart with the head of the cart elevated to approximately 90°. Because normal swallowing usually occurs toward the beginning of exhalation, it is helpful to present food to the patient during the radiographic study at the beginning of the exhalation phase of the respiratory cycle. Often, patients on a ventilator complain that their swallowing worsened when they went onto the ventilator. Swallowing and respiration are reciprocal. Since the ventilator controls the respiratory cycle, the patient cannot lengthen the exhalation to allow for the swallow. If the patient has a slightly slow oral or pharyngeal swallow, which cannot be completed in the time period allocated for exhalation by the ventilator, the swallow may be further disrupted by the restart of inhalation. Also, ventilator-dependant patients normally have a tracheostomy in place with the cuff inflated. The inflated cuff on the tracheostomy may reduce laryngeal elevation and thus reduce closure of the entrance of the airway, which in turn may allow food to enter or penetrate the entrance of the airway and be aspirated after the swallow. Many of these patients can use the Mendelsohn maneuver, the supraglottic swallow, or the supersupraglottic swallow. The Mendelsohn maneuver improves laryngeal elevation, while the supraglottic swallow improves airway closure at the vocal folds or, if done with effort (as in the supersupraglottic swallow), at the entrance to the airway. In either case, since both maneuvers extend the duration of airway closure and thus extend the apneic pause during the swallow, the alarm on the ventilator may sound when the patient is practicing either swallowing maneuver. This will need to be adjusted by nursing or respiratory therapy, if appropriate for a particular patient.

Patients with Cerebral Palsy and Other Movement Disorders

Patients with cerebral palsy and other movement disorders will have difficulty controlling excess movement in their head, neck, and upper body during the swallowing study and during each swallow. This can make visualization of the oral cavity and pharynx during the swallow more difficult. Several alternative techniques can be used to collect information on oropharyngeal swallowing in these patients. First, the patient can be observed during swallows without X ray to see the pattern of head movement during each swallow. Most, though not all, such patients move their head and upper body in a particular pattern during a swallow. Some patients go into extension, while others move forward. If the fluoroscopic tube is positioned so that it views the patients as they are producing the pharyngeal swallow, data on the physiology of this swallowing stage can be collected. The oral stage will not be visualized, as the patients will be positioned out of range of the fluoroscopic tube. However, physiologically, the pharyngeal stage is most critical and it is the stage that cannot be assessed at the bedside with any accuracy. Thus, it is worthwhile to miss the oral stage if the pharyngeal physiology can be viewed.

It is not possible to follow the patient's movement with the fluoroscopic tube. The oropharyngeal swallow is too rapid and human reaction time too slow to move the fluoroscopic tube fast enough to "follow" or adjust for the patient's head or body movement, even if the pattern of movement is anticipated.

A second way to manage excess movement involves stabilizing the patient, usually in a reclining, semireclining, or side-lying position, whichever is most appropriate for a given patient. Most patients with movement disorders are stabilized by their body weight and gravity when they are lying down. Thus, if the previously described technique is not successful, the patient may be put into a side-lying or partially reclining position in order to reduce head-and-neck movement during the radiographic study. This type of positioning is less advantageous because it no longer resembles the patient's normal eating position. However, if the patient's head-and-body movements are random and cannot be anticipated during the swallow, having the patient lie down does allow collection of basic information on the physiology of the oral and pharyngeal stages of the swallow. What is lost is information on how gravity affects bolus flow while the patient is in his or her normal posture for eating. However, data on the physiology of the oropharyngeal stages of the swallow can be collected, and often the effect of gravity can be predicted, once the basic physiology is understood. Positioning the patient in a side-lying or recumbent position is favored over keeping the patient in an upright position and missing the swallow because of excess random movement of the head and upper body. In some cases, laying the child or adult back at a 15° angle from vertical may be sufficient to stabilize the head and upper body to permit good-quality physiologic information to be collected. If possible, the clinician referring the patient should anticipate these kinds of positioning difficulties and recommend optimal positioning during the radiographic study for a child or adult with cerebral palsy or other movement disorders.

Throughout the radiographic study, positioning that reduces excess muscle tone is also desirable. If a wheelchair or other chair puts a child in a better position to reduce excess muscle tone, it should be used during the radiographic study.

Apraxic Patients

Patients with oral apraxia often display swallowing apraxia. This disorder is characterized by a normal range of motion in oral structures but difficulty in initiating and organizing oral movements to produce a normally coordinated oral stage of swallowing when a command to swallow is given. For example, patients will have greater difficulty when instructed to swallow by the examiner than when they are observed eating spontaneously. If the apraxic patient has no suspected pharyngeal swallowing impairment, a radiographic study is not needed. However, some patients have a degree of swallowing apraxia and pharyngeal-stage disorders, such as multistroke patients and certain head-injured patients. If a patient is known to have oral apraxia, the clinician is often most successful in the radiographic examination when no commands to swallow are given. Often, it is best if food is simply placed in the mouth and the patient is given time to swallow. Or patients may be handed the spoon containing food so that they can place it in their mouth themselves. A third alternative is to give patients a dish of food and a spoon and allow them to feed themselves, turning on the fluoroscopy image when food enters their mouth. If none of these techniques facilitate oral initiation and the oral stage of swallowing, additional sensory input may be helpful. Placing food in the mouth with greater downward pressure of the spoon against the tongue, introducing cold food, introducing food requiring chewing, or performing thermal-tactile stimulation prior to food being placed in the mouth for the swallow may all facilitate more normal oral movement and initiation of the swallow.

Visually Impaired Patients

Visually impaired patients, including those with visual-field abnormalities, may not be able to see the food as it is being presented and may become frightened. If patients have visual-field restrictions, it is best to try to present food on the side where they can see most easily. It is also helpful to let the patients feel the empty spoon on their hand and then in their mouth before food is presented. Touching the spoon containing food to a patient's lip before it enters the mouth can provide important sensory alerting. It also is usually helpful to describe the taste as food is being presented.

Infants and Young Children

A number of variations in the MBS procedure previously described may be necessary when examining infants and young children (Morris, 1982). Overall, it is best to position them with minimal fuss and to present foods and liquids as normally as possible. Asking a parent or other caregiver to feed the child may reduce the child's anxiety and give the clinician an opportunity to observe the parent's feeding approach, including such factors as the amount given and placement in the mouth. Usually, the duration of the radiographic study should be kept shorter with the child than with the adult, with the goal of only 2 min of X-ray exposure.

Positioning. Parents or nursing staff (if the child is an inpatient) should be asked to bring the child's usual feeding chair or wheelchair so that optimum positioning can be attained during the radiographic study. If the patient is an infant, the chair can often be set on the platform attached to the fluoroscopy table, or it can be set on a cart, which is then wheeled in and positioned between the fluoroscopy tube and the table (see Figure 4.11). When seated in his or her own chair, the child will generally be more stable and comfortable and more cooperative. Alternatively, the child may be placed in a Tumble Form Feeder Seat on the cart, as shown in Figure 4.11, or laid on the cart and propped in place by pillows. In general, it is best to avoid lifting and moving the child around a great deal, as this can upset the child and a less reliable study will be achieved. A parent or other caregiver should not be allowed to hold the child during the radiographic study, as this will expose them to unneeded radiation.

Desensitization for acceptance of food. Before giving the infant or young child any material to swallow, the clinician should tell the child in simple terms that he or she will be given something to eat. The empty implement to be used in presenting the material (e.g., the spoon) should be held upright within the child's vision to indicate that it contains no food. Prior to placing the implement in the child's mouth, it is sometimes helpful to "desensitize" any oral hypersensitivity by lightly touching the rounded side of the spoon against the lateral aspect of the infant's jaw, near the ear. Light contact should be repeated across the lower edge of the jaw, across to the other side of the face, and back again just under the lip. Each time the light contact is made, the clinician should repeatedly say, "I'm just going to touch," in a soft, reassuring voice. The light contact and verbal comment should be repeated with the spoon under the lip, gradually inching toward the lip. This reduces the patient's fear. The usual response of infants and young children is to slowly open their mouth to accept the empty spoon. The clinician can then place a small amount (1 ml) of liquid on the spoon and slowly introduce it to the oral cavity. Patients should be given time to open their mouth in response to the presentation of food. This procedure of desensitization can be used with adult patients as well if they are functioning at a low cognitive level. Often these patients retract from a spoon as it is brought to their mouth. This physical retraction from food indicates fear and the patient's attempt at self-protection. The clinician should never fight a patient (infant or adult) to place food in his or her mouth.

This process of desensitization is especially helpful for infants and young children who have never been fed by mouth, and who may need to become comfortable with a strange object approaching and entering their mouth. A child should never be

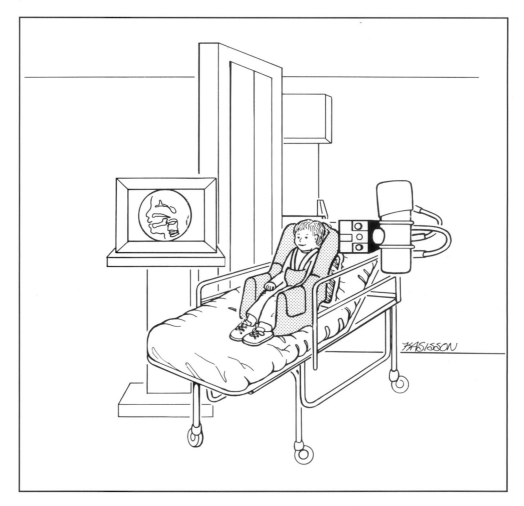

FIGURE 4.11. A drawing illustrating the positioning of an infant or child in a Tumble Form Feeder Seat on a cart in the fluoroscopic suite.

evaluated when crying or fighting the feeding. This only reinforces the child's already negative feelings about feeding. Crying will significantly change swallowing physiology and greatly increase the chances of aspiration.

Selection and presentation of food. Food should be presented with the implement that is most comfortable for the child. If bottle-feeding is used, the parents or nurse should be asked to bring an empty bottle and a bottle of formula. Then a small amount of liquid barium can be mixed with the formula in the empty bottle for presentation to the child. Usually a balance of one-third barium liquid and two-thirds formula will give good radiographic contrast while retaining the flavor of the formula. If the child is eating prepared baby foods or pureed foods, the parents may bring a bottle or small amount of the child's favorite foods, to which a small amount of barium can be added. Again, a balance of two-thirds baby food and one-third barium provides optimum contrast and flavor.

If the patient is a young infant or multiply handicapped child, a parent or familiar clinician may be more successful in presenting the food to the child than the swallowing therapist in Radiology. When this is true, the parent should be given a lead apron and a lead-lined glove to wear in presenting the food, unless the parent's hand is outside the field of X-ray exposure.

Head-Injured Patients

When performing a radiographic study on a head-injured patient, the first problem is often positioning the patient. Adequate seating devices must be available to enable patients with various paretic involvements to be positioned in the radiographic equipment. A number of seating devices for this purpose are now on the market (see Appendix A). If the patient is functioning at a low cognitive level, introduction of food to the oral cavity may require desensitization, as described in the section on infants and children.

During the radiographic study, if the head-injured patient's dysphagic symptoms do not match swallowing physiology, particularly if the patient has chronic copious secretions and no aspiration is seen during the oropharyngeal study, the clinician should proceed to examine the patient for the potential of a tracheoesophageal (TE) fistula. Occasionally, patients with head injury will sustain an injury directly to the chest that penetrates the esophagus, creating a TE fistula. Or the head-injured patient who has been intubated for long periods of time may develop a TE fistula if the end of the tube wears a hole in the common wall between the trachea and esophagus. Whenever a head-injured patient's bedside swallowing symptoms appear worse than his or her actual swallowing physiology during videofluoroscopy, the clinician should consider the possibility that a TE fistula may be present. To search for a TE fistula during X ray, the clinician should lower the fluoroscopic tube to the region of the base of the neck and the top of the chest, that is, the mediastinal area. The clinician should rotate the patient's shoulders at a diagonal, with the head still in a lateral view. With the fluoroscopic tube focused on the mediastinal area of the esophagus and set on magnification, the clinician can give the patient additional food to be swallowed and look for a TE fistula. The fistula will appear as food progresses through the esophagus, reaches the fistula, and passes into the trachea. A TE fistula is not common in head-injured patients, but it does occur in a small percentage of these patients.

Head-injured patients should be reevaluated at regular intervals to assess objectively their recovery toward normal oropharyngeal swallow (Ylvisaker & Logemann, 1986). Even those patients in whom recovery is slow or appears to be extremely limited should be reassessed. We repeatedly see head-injured individuals for whom long-term nonoral feeding is given and swallowing therapy is terminated because of lack of progress, who then return a year or two later with normal swallowing. Clearly, we do not understand enough about swallowing rehabilitation and spontaneous recovery of swallowing after head injury to predict accurately which head-injured patients will recover and which will not. Careful assessment of the oropharyngeal stages of swallowing, both physiologic and clinical, provides the best opportunity for the patient's recovery of swallowing, when this assessment is followed by appropriate therapy and management.

Mentally Retarded or Developmentally Delayed Patients

Individuals with mental retardation or developmental delay often behave like infants and young children in the radiographic study. That is, they localize to any sound and are fearful of strange, unfamiliar situations. Often it is helpful to bring such individuals into the radiographic suite a day or two before the scheduled radiographic study to show them the equipment and acclimate them to the surroundings. It is also helpful to let them hear the sounds made by the videofluoroscopic equipment. Allowing these patients to see the video screen or hold a toy or familiar object can be helpful in distracting them during the study. All of the procedures described earlier for infants and young children are applicable to the mentally retarded or developmentally delayed population.

Variations in Food Presentation

Consistency of Food Presented

In some instances the clinician will want to modify the food consistencies given to a patient during the MBS procedure. Specifically, the patient is usually given food of three consistencies in small amounts, as described earlier: liquid, paste, and material to be masticated (cookie). If a patient has no teeth, the cookie may be omitted. Instead the clinician may wish to provide the patient with food of an intermediate consistency between liquid and the heavy paste—something similar to a thick milkshake. To reach this consistency, the clinician can simply mix the liquid and thick paste until the desired consistency is achieved.

If a patient complains of swallowing difficulty with a particular type of food, or with material such as meat or medications, the clinician may wish to give the patient this type of food and examine any differences that occur in swallowing control. However, care should be taken when giving barium tablets or capsules, as they may become lodged in the pharynx or esophagus or fall into the airway.

Some clinicians recommend using a larger variety of food consistencies, perhaps 6 or 10, in the radiographic study. When expanding the number of consistencies used, the clinician should always weigh the information to be gained against the additional radiation exposure for the patient, particularly if the patient's swallowing function is to be reassessed later.

Flavor of Food Presented

Bedside introduction of various flavors may identify a particular flavor that appears to elicit faster or more efficient oral or pharyngeal swallowing. If so, this flavor should be introduced to the patient in the radiographic study and compared with swallows of the same volume and consistency in which this flavor is not used.

Order of Food Presentation

At times, the clinician will want to begin the MBS with food of a consistency other than liquid. With young children who are uncooperative, the clinician may wish to begin with the chocolate pudding mixed with barium or with a small piece of cookie, which looks more appetizing than the liquid barium compound.

Occasionally, a severely impaired head trauma patient will not respond when liquid or paste is placed in his or her mouth. That is, no tongue movement will be initiated to manipulate the food or start a swallow. This food will need to be suctioned or wiped from the mouth. Some of these patients will respond, however, when food of a heavier consistency requiring mastication, such as a cookie, is placed in their mouth. When these patients are given the piece of cookie, they often begin to chew spontaneously and will then initiate a swallow. Occasionally such patients will begin chewing and will continue chewing without ever initiating a swallow.

Amount of Food Presented

In many radiographic studies, the clinician will wish to increase the amount of food given to the patient. If a patient does not initiate a pharyngeal swallow at all on the first few 1-ml liquid swallows, the amount given to the patient may be increased to 3 ml to see if the larger volume will improve the triggering of the pharyngeal swallow. In some patients, increasing the volume results in faster triggering of the pharyngeal swallow.

Patients with reduced tongue control but good laryngeal airway protection will need to "dump" large amounts of material into the pharynx quickly to be able to get sufficient nutrition by mouth. Before the clinician attempts this feeding technique at the bedside, it should be attempted and assessed on fluoroscopy. In this case, the clinician can give the patient ⅓ cup of barium and ask him or her to take as much as is desired, as fast as is desired. This should only be done when the patient has clearly demonstrated timely triggering of the pharyngeal swallow and good airway protection, but poor tongue control on previous swallows of smaller amounts. This method of feeding requires that the patient keep his or her airway closed while literally dumping material into the pharynx and repeatedly swallowing to clear the material, without breathing between swallows (an extended supraglottic swallow). After the repeated swallows, the patient must cough and clear his or her throat to remove any residue from the opening into the airway. Performing this procedure during fluoroscopy documents that the patient can get a sufficient amount of food down quickly enough to maintain nutrition without significant aspiration. It also allows the clinician to provide the patient with feedback regarding when and how effortfully to cough in order to expectorate the residual material successfully from the top of the airway.

If the patient is feeding by taking in larger amounts of food per bolus and drinking from a cup and has a history of pneumonia, excessive congestion, pulmonary problems, or coughing or choking when swallowing, and if the MBS using small amounts of material has revealed a normal swallow, the clinician should try to simulate normal feeding procedures and examine them radiographically. It may be that the patient can handle small amounts of food per bolus but has physiologic problems handling larger amounts. These differences should then be studied.

Method of Food Presentation

At times, the clinician will need to use special implements to present the food to the patient because of the patient's particular anatomic or physiologic impairments. Normally, 1 ml and 3 ml of liquid, paste, and piece of cookie can be presented on a spoon, whereas 5 ml and 10 ml of liquid can be measured and presented to the lips and front of the mouth in a syringe or an empty cup. If the patient cannot open his or her mouth widely, has a tongue thrust, or has reduced tongue tissue or tongue movement to propel food backward, the clinician may need to present material to the back of the mouth in a syringe. A 1-ml syringe is usually best. It is narrow in diameter (¼ in.) and is just long enough so that when the tip of the syringe is positioned over the back of the tongue, as shown in Figure 4.12, the rim of the syringe is at the lips. In this way food will drop into the pharynx and will not fall back toward the front of the mouth. When using a syringe, the patient should be able to protect his or her airway.

Otherwise, food squirted into the pharynx may fall directly into the airway. Only a small amount of liquid (⅓ ml) should be given until airway protection has been demonstrated.

A Mothercare spoon may also be used to present material to patients who have a narrow mouth opening or who have a tendency to trigger a bite reflex. These spoons have a very shallow bowl and are made of heavy-duty plastic, so they do not break in response to a bite reflex.

In patients with poor tongue control but normal soft palate function, a straw may be positioned far back in the mouth in such a way that the end of the straw is held between the back of the tongue and the palate. In this way the oral phase of the swallow can be bypassed. A straw may also be used as a pipette to position a small amount of liquid in a specific spot in the oral cavity.

Occasionally, as described earlier, a cup may be used to present larger amounts of liquid. Patients can hold their breath to close the airway (supraglottic swallow), tilt their head back, and drop material into the pharynx in much the same way as with a syringe. If patients initially use a syringe to bypass the oral phase of the swallow, it is usually best to attempt to advance them to a cup so that they can eat in a more socially acceptable manner. With infants and young children, a bottle may be used to present liquid.

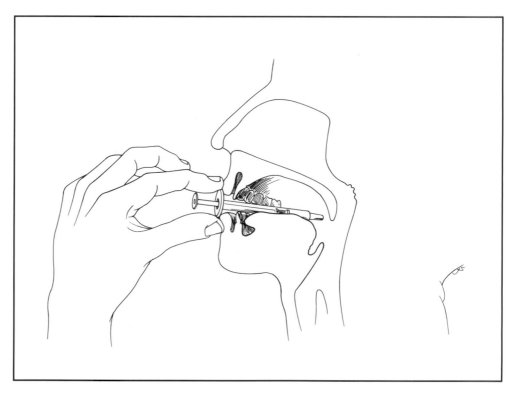

FIGURE 4.12.   A lateral view of the oral cavity, with a 1-ml syringe positioned posteriorly in the oral cavity.

Special-Purpose Tests

Fatiguing the Patient

If a patient complains of difficulty swallowing and the MBS is normal, the clinician may wish to fatigue the patient to rule out myasthenia gravis or general fatiguing as an etiology. Myasthenia gravis can affect any muscles innervated by cranial nerves, including the musculature of the tongue, soft palate, larynx, or pharynx (Aronson, 1981; Logemann, 1983). Symptoms of myasthenia gravis come with fatigue. Thus, if there is reason to suspect that the patient may show changes in swallowing with muscle fatigue, the patient should be examined twice. After the first MBS study is completed, the patient should continue to eat or be fed for 15 or 20 min. After eating, the patient's swallowing should again be evaluated radiographically. During the MBS, the patient should be given liquid in a glass and asked to take five or six continuous swallows. This "fatigue study" is likely to reveal any symptoms of myasthenia gravis.

Assessing Spasm Versus Stricture in Total Laryngectomees

Stricture is an anatomic abnormality (narrowing) that can occur in total laryngectomees. If present, it restricts the passage of the bolus through the pharyngoesophagus. A stricture is visible and present at all times during swallowing and voice production. During swallowing, a stricture is seen as a narrowed region, above which food collects. A spasm in total laryngectomees is a functional contraction in muscles in the pharyngoesophagus in response to the attempt to introduce or release airflow into or out of the esophagus. A spasm is not present during swallowing but is present during voice attempts. Therefore, during the radiographic study of swallowing and speech in total laryngectomees, swallowing assessment should be completed first. If stricture is present, the bolus will collect in the pharyngoesophagus and not flow freely. Swallowing will coat the pharyngoesophagus with barium. The stricture will also be present on voice attempts. After the swallow, esophageal voice attempts can be observed radiographically and an air-blowing test can be performed. If a bar or obstruction to air intake or release is observed on voice attempts and not on swallowing, a spasm is present.

Modifications in Viewing Structural Detail

Several modifications can be made in examining the patient that facilitate assessment of anatomic structures.

Magnification

Most fluoroscopy machines are capable of magnifying the image to assess particular anatomic areas in the head-and-neck region more carefully. For example, if there is some particular question about vocal fold function, the top of the airway may be magnified so that, in an anterior view, the movement patterns of the vocal folds can be evaluated more closely. Or the cricopharyngeal–upper esophageal juncture may be viewed more closely. Magnification is particularly useful in examination of infants in order to view the pharynx more easily.

Still Radiographs

At any time during the MBS, still radiographs may be taken to record the hesitation of the bolus, the amount and location of residue, or the relationship of anatomic structures. It must always be remembered, however, that any still radiograph represents only a single instant in time and must be interpreted carefully. The clinician must be sure to note the particular moment during the swallow when the picture was taken. Also, because taking a still radiograph will interrupt the fluoroscopic image momentarily, still radiographs should not be taken during critical events in the swallow.

Videoprints

Videoprinters will produce a print of any single video image held in the pause mode on the video screen. This enables the clinician to make a copy of any single event during the swallow, even if it is visible for only a fraction of a second. Videoprints are made from the completed radiographic study rather than during the study, as still radiographs are made.

Summary

Variations on the standard MBS, can expand the value of the test. The clinician can verify (a) the validity of particular changes in posture and other therapy procedures in terms of their effects on the clearance of food and presence or elimination of aspiration, (b) the effects of changing the food consistency or the order of foods given, (c) the effects of larger amounts of material, and (d) the impact of changing the method of food presentation.

To use these variations on the standard procedure, the clinician must be able to "read" the results of each swallow immediately during the MBS procedure. In the clinician's early experience with the technique, this may not be accomplished easily. That is, the clinician may not be able to apply the variations on the MBS procedure until he or she has become highly experienced in quickly reading the X-ray studies. In this case, the clinician may wish to complete the swallow-assessment portion of the test, read the X ray later, and schedule the treatment portion of the test for a different day. It is important that the clinician not simply apply at random all of the procedural variations previously described. Instead, the variations must be applied selectively and should be given only to patients with the particular swallowing problems for which each variation in procedure is appropriate.

The videotapes of the MBS and its procedural variations can be used for education of physicians, other health care professionals, and the patient and family so that they can better understand the rationales for the clinician's use of particular compensatory techniques or therapy strategies. Often, families are overanxious to feed a patient because they cannot see any external signs of swallowing difficulty; for example, the patient may not cough or choke visibly. Well-meaning families and friends will usually reduce their attempts at feeding when they can see the actual abnormal physiology of the patient's swallows and the effectiveness of the particular postures and other therapy procedures.

Radiographic Symptoms and Swallowing Disorders

Interpretation of the radiographic assessment of oropharyngeal swallowing involves observing movement of the bolus in relation to movement of the structures of the mouth and pharynx. Movement of the bolus can be measured in terms of duration of movement through the mouth (oral transit time) and pharynx (pharyngeal transit time). Efficiency of bolus movement can be described in terms of the location and approximate amount of residual food in the mouth and pharynx. Safety of food movement can be defined according to whether or not any food enters (penetrates) the airway entrance down to the level of the surface of the vocal folds or when and how much food enters the airway below the vocal folds (is aspirated). In addition, the range of movement of structures in the mouth and pharynx can be measured.

Aspiration and residue are symptoms of swallowing disorders, not disorders themselves. Therefore, in this chapter, symptoms are related to the swallowing disorders that cause them. The chapter and the accompanying videofluorographic worksheet (Appendix B) are organized to parallel the MBS procedure. Thus, the radiographic symptoms of swallowing disorders that may be observed in the oral preparatory, oral, pharyngeal, and cervical esophageal stages of the swallow in the lateral view are described first and listed first on the worksheet. The last third of the chapter and the worksheet present the symptoms of swallowing disorders that may be observed in the oral preparatory and pharyngeal stages of the swallow when viewed in the P-A plane.

On the worksheet, the far right-hand column identifies swallowing disorders, while the far left-hand column presents symptoms. That is, the symptoms or observations noted on the left are indicative of particular swallowing disorders, which are noted in the far right-hand column. For example, residue in the pharynx, particularly on the pharyngeal walls and in the pyriform sinus on only one side (as listed in the left-hand column), would be an indication of unilateral dysfunction of the pharyngeal wall (listed in the right-hand column). Residue of food in the lateral sulcus in the oral cavity (noted in the left column) is an indication of reduced tension in the buccal musculature (noted in the right column). Thus, residue in the lateral sulcus is a radiographic symptom listed in the left-hand column under the oral stage of swallowing, while reduced buccal tension is the swallowing disorder causing the symptom and is listed in the far right-hand column. The swallowing disorders listed in the right-hand column that relate to the radiographic symptoms in the left-hand column are meant to act as reminders to the clinician of the possible meaning of the symptoms seen radiographically. This list of includes the most common symptoms and disorders; however, it is not meant to be exhaustive, but rather to serve as a guide to clinicians in assessing

73

the videofluoroscopic studies. Disorders other than those listed on the worksheet may occasionally be seen. If so, there is room at the end of each swallowing stage on the worksheet to note other disorders (in the column marked "Other") as they occur on the various volumes and consistencies.

The Lateral View

The lateral view permits examination and measurement of oral and pharyngeal transit times; movement patterns of the bolus and oropharyngeal structures in the oral preparatory, oral, pharyngeal, and cervical esophageal aspects of deglutition; and the amount and cause (etiology) of any aspiration that occurs. Oral transit time (OTT) is defined as the time taken from the initiation of the tongue movement that begins the voluntary oral stage of the swallow until the pharyngeal swallow (swallowing reflex) is triggered (Miller, 1982; Pommerenke, 1928). Normally, this time is approximately 1 to 1.25 sec (Mandelstam & Lieber, 1970; Tracy et al., 1989). Pharyngeal transit time (PTT) is defined as the time elapsed from the moment when the bolus head passes the point where the shadow of the mandible crosses the base of the tongue (see Figure 5.12) until the bolus tail passes through the cricopharyngeal region or the pharyngoesophageal segment. This time is normally a maximum of 1 sec, usually far less (0.35 to 0.48 sec) (Blonsky et al., 1978; Mandelstam & Lieber, 1970; Tracy et al., 1989).

The lateral view of the oral cavity, pharynx, and larynx also facilitates the observation of whether or not aspiration occurs, estimation of the percentage of aspiration, and determination of the cause of the aspiration. In the P-A view, the trachea and the esophagus overlap each other, and it is difficult to assess the amount of aspiration and its cause. It is critical to note whether aspiration occurs before, during, or after the pharyngeal swallow and to identify the physiologic or anatomic causal factors for the aspiration. Treatment is then designed to eradicate the aspiration by eliminating its etiology.

Disorders in Oral Preparation of the Swallow

The oral preparatory stage of the swallow is designed to break food down into an appropriate consistency for the swallow and mix it with saliva. A number of disorders can be identified in the lateral view during oral preparation for the swallow. Some disorders in this phase, however, must be examined in the P-A view. These will be discussed later.

Cannot hold food in the mouth anteriorly—reduced lip closure. Normally, as food is placed in the mouth, the lips close and remain closed during all phases of the swallow to keep food in the mouth anteriorly. When food falls from the mouth anteriorly, it is an indication of reduced lip closure, as shown in Figure 5.1.

Cannot form a bolus—reduced range of tongue motion or coordination. During mastication, or while the patient is merely tasting material in the mouth prior to the swallow, food is normally manipulated and moved throughout the oral cavity. When the individual is finished with mastication or oral manipulation, food is pulled together by the tongue into a single ball or bolus to initiate the swallow. If a patient has a reduced range or coordination of tongue movement, he or she will have difficulty in pulling this food back together into a cohesive bolus, and thus will often be forced to initiate a swallow with food spread throughout the oral cavity.

Cannot hold a bolus—reduced tongue shaping and coordination. Liquid and paste materials are placed into the oral cavity as a cohesive or semicohesive bolus. Normally, unless an individual wants to taste material or otherwise manipulate it in the mouth, the liquid or paste is kept in a cohesive bolus, or ball, awaiting the initia-

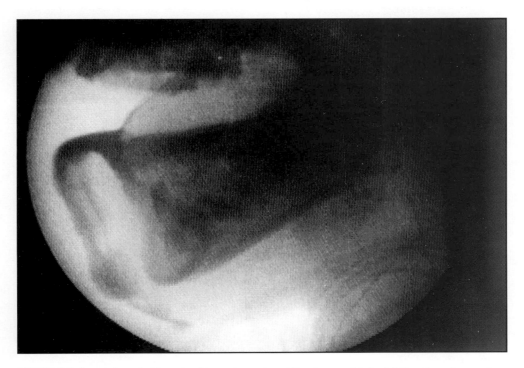

FIGURE 5.1. A lateral videoprint illustrating reduced lip closure with food falling from the mouth and over the lower lip.

tion of the oral phase of the swallow. If a patient has reduced ability to shape the tongue around the liquid or paste, he or she will be unable to hold the liquid or paste in a cohesive bolus, and material will immediately spread throughout the oral cavity. If the soft palate cannot or does not bulge anteriorly to contact the back of the tongue, food can be lost into the pharynx prematurely. Premature loss of bolus over the tongue base and into the pharynx is normal during mastication but not while holding a liquid bolus. This can result in aspiration before the swallow if the liquid or food falls over the base of the tongue into the pharynx and the open airway.

Whether or not aspiration will occur depends upon the amount of food given, its consistency, and the exact posture of the patient. Inability to hold a bolus is an indication of reduced tongue coordination. Premature loss into the valleculae on liquid or paste is an indication of reduced anterior soft palate positioning.

Material falls into anterior sulcus—reduced labial tension or tone. Food falling into the anterior sulcus, after it has been placed in the oral cavity or as the patient is chewing, is an indication of reduced labial or facial muscle tone. Muscle tone in the labial and facial musculature is responsible for closing the anterior sulcus and preventing food from lodging there.

Material falls into lateral sulcus—reduced buccal tension or tone. Material falling into the lateral sulcus as the patient chews is an indication of reduced muscle tension or tone in the buccal musculature, as shown in Figure 5.2. Normally, tension or tone in the buccal musculature closes the lateral sulcus and prevents material from lodging there by directing it medially toward the tongue.

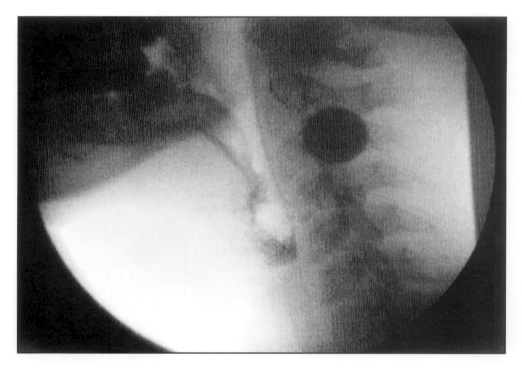

FIGURE 5.2.   A lateral videoprint illustrating material remaining in the lateral sulcus.

Abnormal hold position—tongue thrust; reduced tongue control. Normally, the bolus is held between the tongue and the hard palate in preparation for the initiation of the oral phase of the swallow, or on the floor of the mouth in front of the tongue tip. If the bolus is held on the floor of the mouth, the tongue picks it up and brings it onto the tongue. Approximately 20% of normal subjects exhibit this pattern of bolus hold, which is often seen in older adults (Dodds et al., 1989). To hold and pick up the bolus, the tongue must be able to shape itself around the bolus and seal the sides of the tongue to the lateral alveolar ridge. If tongue shaping is not possible, the patient may hold the bolus in an abnormal position. If the bolus is held against the front teeth, as seen in Figure 5.3, it is likely that the swallow will be accomplished with a tongue-thrusting behavior (i.e., a forward movement of the tongue toward the lips and central incisors that pushes the bolus forward). Often this tongue thrust is so strong that it actually pushes the food out of the oral cavity. As described here, this tongue thrust relates to neurologic impairment and is seen in some patients with cerebral palsy and in some individuals after stroke or head trauma.

Other. This space is provided for the clinician to note any other abnormal movement patterns that may be observed during the oral preparatory phase of the swallow in the lateral view.

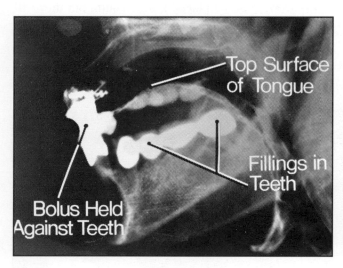

FIGURE 5.3. A lateral radiograph illustrating an abnormal hold position of the bolus against the front teeth.

Disorders in the Oral Phase of Deglutition

The oral phase of deglutition consists of lingual propulsion of the bolus through the oral cavity. This phase of the swallow is considered to be under voluntary control, but it plays a role in the initiation (triggering) of the pharyngeal swallow. The oral phase of the swallow begins when the front of the tongue initiates backward movement of the bolus with an upward and backward motion of the midline of the tongue, and terminates when the pharyngeal swallow is triggered (Kahrilas et al., in press; Shawker, Sonies, Stone, & Baum, 1983). The pharyngeal swallow is normally triggered anywhere from the anterior faucial arch to the base of the tongue and valleculae via sensory input to (predominantly) the ninth cranial nerve (i.e., the glossopharyngeal nerve). The total OTT in normal individuals is approximately 1 to 1.25 sec for all consistencies of material swallowed (Mandelstam & Lieber, 1970; Tracy et al., 1989).

Delayed oral onset of swallow—apraxia of swallow; reduced oral sensation. Some severely neurologically impaired patients exhibit significant delay in initiating the oral swallow when given a swallowing command. Often the bolus is held in the mouth with no lingual movement, as shown in Figure 5.4. This symptom may indicate a severe swallowing apraxia, reduced oral sensation, or lack of recognition of the bolus as something to be swallowed. Increasing sensory stimulation for these patients by increasing the pressure of the spoon on the tongue or using a cold bolus or a textured bolus may cause the oral swallow to begin (see Chapter 4). Also, some of these patients will not react to liquid or pureed material placed in the mouth, but they will begin chewing in response to a small piece of cookie and, after the chewing, will begin the oral swallow.

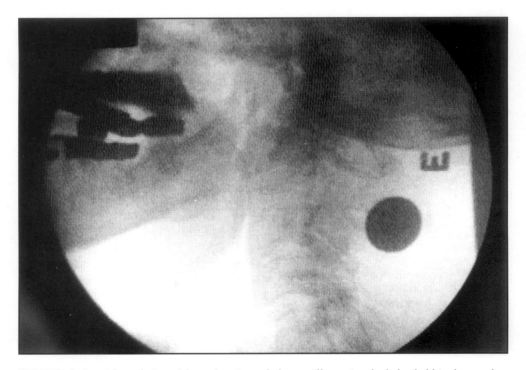

FIGURE 5.4.   A lateral view of the oral cavity and pharynx illustrating the bolus held in the mouth during the hesitation in initiating the oral swallow.

Searching motion; inability to organize tongue movements—apraxia of swallow. Apraxia of swallow usually accompanies severe oral apraxia. Symptoms of swallowing apraxia include making searching movements with the tongue, exhibiting good range of motion but inability to organize the front-to-back lingual movement with the bolus associated with a swallow, or, in some cases, simply holding the bolus without initiating any oral activity (Robbins & Levine, 1988). Increasing sensory stimulation as the bolus is presented or giving a bolus that has a distinct temperature, flavor, or texture may facilitate organized tongue movement during the oral swallow. Also, presenting the bolus to patients on a spoon and allowing them to place the bolus in their mouth themselves or giving them the food and spoon to feed themselves normally may facilitate oral activity. Refraining from giving any commands to swallow can also be helpful, since apraxia is usually worse when the target activity becomes highly volitional.

Tongue moves forward to start the swallow—tongue thrust. Normally, when the bolus is on the tongue, the tongue tip remains anchored against the alveolar ridge and initiates the swallow by lifting the front and center in the midline upward and backward against the palate. Neurologic impairment may cause the tongue to thrust forward toward the central incisors, sometimes pushing food from the mouth as shown in Figure 5.5. Usually, a tongue thrust is preceded by an abnormal hold position of the bolus against the central incisors or an inability to hold the bolus at all, as is seen in some individuals with cerebral palsy.

Residue (stasis) in the anterior sulcus—reduced labial tension or tone. If, during initiation of the oral phase of the swallow, the bolus lodges in the anterior sulcus, it is a symptom of reduced labial-buccal muscle tension or tone and poor lingual control.

Residue (stasis) in the lateral sulcus—reduced buccal muscle tension or tone. If, during initiation of the oral phase of the swallow, food falls or lodges in the lateral sulcus, as shown in Figure 5.2, it is an indication of reduced muscle tension or tone in

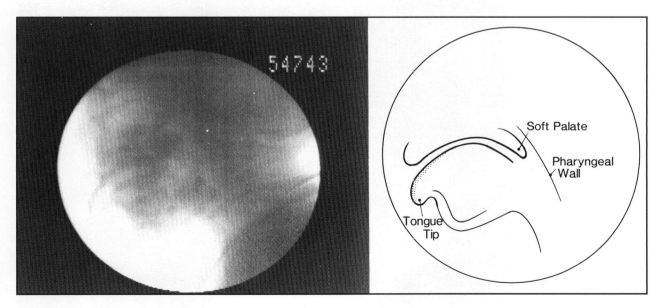

FIGURE 5.5. A lateral videoprint illustrating a tongue thrust in a child with cerebral palsy. The tongue is protruding from the mouth approximately 1 1/2 in.

the buccal musculature. Some investigators believe that buccal muscle tension plays a role in the backward movement of the bolus during oral transit by providing resistance or pressure in the lateral walls of the oral cavity (Shedd, Scatliff, & Kirchner, 1960).

Residue (stasis) on the floor of the mouth—reduced tongue shaping or coordination. If food falls onto the anterior or lateral floor of the mouth during attempts at oral transit, it is an indication of reduced ability by the patient to shape and coordinate the tongue around the bolus (i.e., to maintain contact of the tongue tip and sides to the alveolus) as it moves posteriorly. Figure 5.6 illustrates residual food on the anterior floor of the mouth in a surgically treated oral cancer patient, while Figure 5.7 illustrates residue on the lateral floor of the mouth in another surgically treated oral cancer patient.

Residue (stasis) in a midtongue depression—scar tissue in tongue. If food tends to lodge in a depression in the tongue's surface, it usually indicates scar tissue in the tongue. Scar tissue can appear quite benign on anatomic examination (i.e., when the speech pathologist or physician does an oral examination of the tongue). However, it is usually tight and relatively immobile; when the patient attempts to swallow, the normal tongue tissue surrounding the scar can elevate and move, but the scar tissue cannot, thus forming a deep crevice into which food will fall as the patient struggles to swallow. The greater the lingual struggle to swallow, the worse the effect of the scar tissue on the swallow will be, and the greater the amount of food that will collect in the depression created by the scar tissue. Figure 5.8 illustrates residue in a midtongue depression in a surgically treated oral cancer patient. When scar tissue is present, it is usually the result of surgical treatment for oral cancer or some trauma to the mouth, such as a knife or gunshot wound.

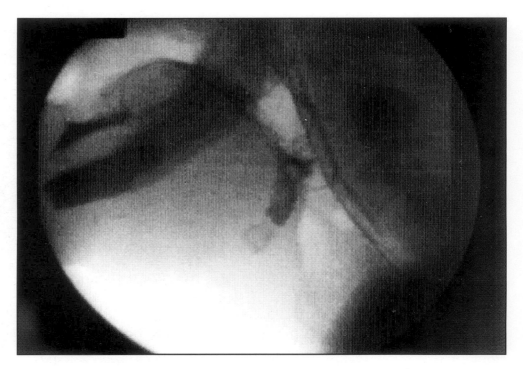

FIGURE 5.6.   A lateral videoprint of a surgically treated oral cancer patient with residue remaining on the anterior floor of the mouth as well as in the valleculae after the swallow.

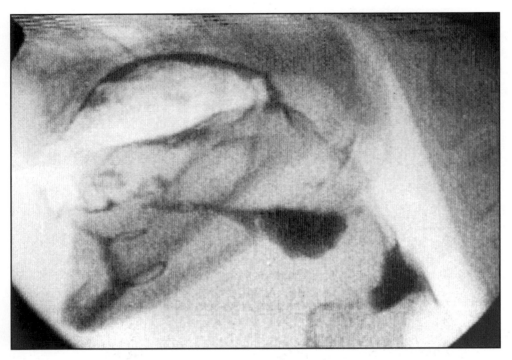

FIGURE 5.7.   A lateral view of the oral cavity and oropharynx illustrating mild residue on the hard palate, moderate residue on the posterior lateral floor of the mouth, and moderate residue in the valleculae.

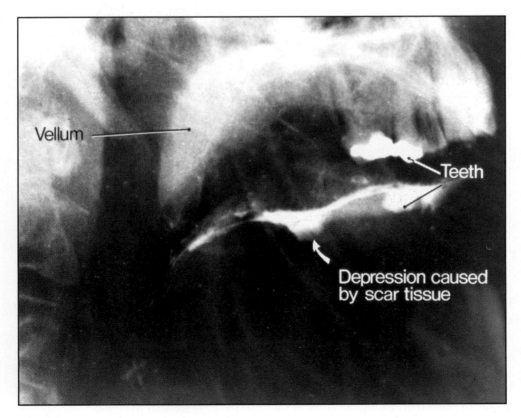

FIGURE 5.8.   A lateral radiograph of the oral cavity in a surgically treated oral cancer patient with scar tissue in the midtongue depression where residual food collects.

Residue (stasis) of food on the tongue—reduced tongue range of movement; reduced tongue strength.   If tongue range of movement is very poor, food may sit on the tongue surface and remain there despite numerous attempts to initiate a swallow. This usually occurs with food of thicker consistency, since liquid will tend to splash around the oral cavity and collect in the natural crevices rather than on the tongue itself. Any stasis or residue of food on the tongue is an indication of reduced tongue range of movement. If the residue increases as food becomes more viscous, it is an indication of reduced tongue strength.

Disturbed lingual contraction (peristalsis)—lingual discoordination.   In normal swallowing, the tongue tip and sides remain in contact with the anterior and lateral alveolar ridge, while the front and center envelop the bolus and then elevate and squeeze or roll the bolus along the hard palate until it reaches the anterior faucial arches. Thus, the midline of the tongue is elevating sequentially while squeezing against the palate. This is done in a single organized action. If this sequential squeezing action is in any way disturbed (e.g., if the tongue moves in somewhat random, nonproductive motions), the normal smooth anterior-to-posterior movement becomes disorganized. This disturbed lingual contraction is to be distinguished from a repetitive kind of tongue movement pattern, such as the repetitive lingual rolling motion often seen in parkinsonian patients, described later.

Incomplete tongue-to-palate contact—reduced tongue elevation.   In the normal initiation of a swallow, sequential front-to-back tongue-to-palate contact is made as the bolus is moved backward. If tongue-palate contact is incomplete, it is an indication of a reduced range of vertical tongue motion. This may also result in disturbances in lingual contraction or in struggling behavior of the tongue. If there is a great deal of lingual struggling action, the bolus may be spread throughout the mouth.

Adherence (residue) of food on the hard palate—reduced tongue elevation; reduced lingual strength.   Normally, as the tongue propels the bolus posteriorly, there is only minimal food residue left coating the oral structures. When food is observed to collect on the hard palate and to remain there after the swallow, it is an indication of reduced tongue elevation. If increased amounts of food collect on the palate as more viscous food is presented, it is an indication of reduced tongue strength, since increased lingual pressure is needed to propel more viscous food. Figure 5.9 illustrates residual food collected on the palate in a patient with motor neuron disease.

Reduced anterior-posterior lingual action—reduced lingual coordination.   Normal lingual propulsion of the bolus involves smooth front-to-back action of the midline of the tongue. If this smooth front-to-back action is interrupted or broken into multiple small tongue movements in the presence of normal range of motion, it is a symptom of reduced lingual coordination.

Repetitive lingual rolling—Parkinson's disease.   In the normal swallow, the midline of the tongue produces a single upward and backward motion, propelling the bolus posteriorly. Parkinsonian patients show a typical tongue movement pattern characterized by a repetitive upward and backward movement of the central portion of the tongue. The posterior tongue, however, fails to lower at the appropriate time, so the bolus can only move to the region of the posterior hard palate before it rolls forward again. The front tongue activity then repeats itself in an attempt to reinitiate the swallow. This repetitive front-to-back rolling motion of the tongue can often be seen to last 10 sec or more before a full swallow is initiated in parkinsonian patients.

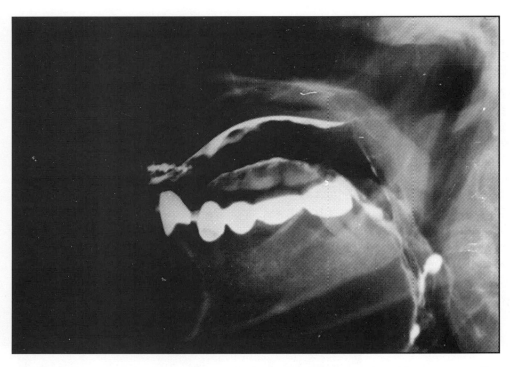

FIGURE 5.9. A lateral videoprint of the oral cavity and pharynx in a patient with motor neuron disease who exhibits residual food on the palate after the swallow.

Uncontrolled bolus or premature loss of liquid or pudding consistency into the pharynx—reduced tongue control; reduced linguavelar seal. An uncontrolled bolus or premature loss of liquid or pudding into the pharynx indicates that during the oral preparatory phase prior to initiation of the oral stage of swallowing, or during the lingual initiation of the swallow, part or all of the bolus has already fallen over the base of the tongue, prematurely, into the pharynx. By definition, this occurs while the oral preparatory or oral stages of swallowing are still under way, prior to the triggering of the pharyngeal swallow. When liquid or pudding boluses are placed in the mouth, the soft palate should be pulled down and anteriorly against the back of the tongue, sealing the bolus in the mouth posteriorly. If this seal fails, part or all of the bolus can be lost into the pharynx prematurely. On foods requiring chewing, premature loss of food into the valleculae is normal, since the contact of the soft palate to the base of the tongue is not maintained because of the chewing motions. Thus, during the radiographic study of the oropharyngeal swallow, if premature loss of bolus is observed on liquid or pudding materials, it is abnormal; but it is not an abnormal behavior during chewing.

When part of the liquid or pudding bolus falls into the pharynx prematurely, it may lodge in the valleculae or the pyriform sinuses, or it may fall into the open airway. The exact path of the food when it lands in the pharynx will depend upon the patient's posture, the amount of food taken, and the consistency of the food. An uncontrolled bolus and premature loss indicate reduced lingual control during the oral preparatory or oral phase of the swallow. This may result in aspiration before the swallow since a part of the bolus is lost into the pharynx before the pharyngeal swallow is triggered and while the airway is open. It is important to note here that the entry of this material into the pharynx does not trigger a pharyngeal swallow. In all probability, no pharyngeal swallow is triggered because the tongue has not yet completed its necessary movement. The patient is barely initiating the oral phase of the swallow when part of the material falls into the pharynx in an uncontrolled manner. Until the tongue propels the remaining bolus to the point where a pharyngeal swallow would be triggered, the mere presence of this material in the pharynx will not trigger the pharyngeal swallow. It may be that this lack of initiation of the pharyngeal swallow in response to material in the pharynx indicates a neurological "priority" system. That is, as long as the patient is still in the oral preparatory or oral phases of the swallow, this voluntary motor activity may neurologically override the sensory input from the food in the pharynx, which might otherwise trigger a pharyngeal swallow. Figure 5.10 illustrates premature loss of a liquid bolus into the pharynx.

If food requiring chewing is given to the patient, premature loss of food into the pharynx (valleculae) is normal. It is most apt to occur when larger amounts of food requiring chewing are placed in the mouth. Premature loss of food is not normal on small (1- to 10-ml) measured amounts of liquid or pudding unless the material is masticated.

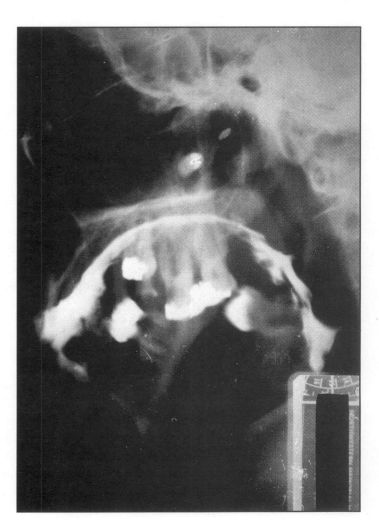

FIGURE 5.10. A lateral videoprint of the oral cavity and pharynx illustrating premature loss of the bolus into the pharynx.

Piecemeal deglutition. The term *piecemeal deglutition* indicates that rather than swallowing the bolus in a single cohesive mass, the patient swallows only one portion or piece of the bolus at a time. Thus the patient requires two, three, or more repeated swallows to empty the oral cavity. This might be normal behavior if the bolus were very large (e.g., 15 ml). But in the MBS, the patient is only given small amounts of food to swallow. These small amounts should be cleared from the oral cavity in a single swallow. Piecemeal deglutition may indicate a fear of swallowing, as the patient carefully meters out small amounts to be swallowed for fear of swallowing an entire bolus and aspirating.

Oral transit time (in seconds). As indicated earlier, OTT in normal individuals should last no more than 1 to 1.25 sec and increases slightly as bolus viscosity increases. In subjects over age 60, oral transit also increases slightly (by approximately 0.25 sec). The reason for slowed OTT should be defined according to the disorder observed in the oral phase of swallow. A slow OTT must be considered in combination with PTT to determine the full duration of the oropharyngeal swallow. The speed of the swallow through the oral and pharyngeal stages is one important factor in determining whether a patient is going to get sufficient nutrition by mouth, as discussed in more detail later in this book (see Chapter 8).

Other. This space is provided for the clinician to note any other abnormal movement patterns or disorders that may be observed during the oral phase of the swallow in the lateral view. Some specific abnormal patterns of tongue movement are characteristic of specific types of patients. These may be noted here.

Postural and treatment techniques introduced to mitigate oral-phase disorders can be noted at the end of this section.

Disorders in Triggering the Pharyngeal Swallow—Transition Between the Oral and Pharyngeal Stages of Swallow

Delayed pharyngeal swallow. Normally, when the head of the bolus passes the tongue base (the point where the lower edge of the mandible crosses the tongue base, as identified on Figures 5.11 and 5.12), the pharyngeal swallow should have begun. Delayed pharyngeal swallow occurs when the head of the bolus enters the pharynx and the pharyngeal swallow has not been triggered, that is, laryngeal elevation in the context of the rest of the pharyngeal swallow has not occurred. The presence of the bolus head below the tongue base in the pharynx increases the risk of aspiration as long as the pharyngeal swallow has not been initiated. Most patients with delay in triggering the pharyngeal swallow complain of difficulty swallowing liquids. Thin liquids are usually swallowed in larger volumes (10 to 20 ml) and will splash into the pharynx rapidly. If the pharyngeal swallow has not been initiated as the liquid passes the tongue base, there is increased risk that the liquid will enter the open airway before the pharyngeal swallow has been activated.

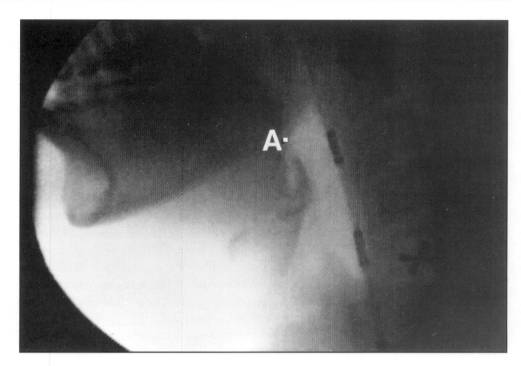

FIGURE 5.11. A lateral videoprint of the oral cavity and pharynx, illustrating the location of the lower edge of the mandible as it crosses the tongue base (*A*), where timing of the triggering of the pharyngeal swallow should begin.

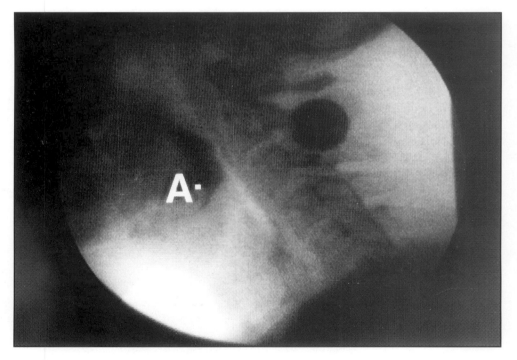

FIGURE 5.12. A lateral radiograph of the oral cavity and pharynx illustrating the location of the point (*A*) where the timing of pharyngeal delay begins.

During a pharyngeal swallow delay, the bolus may land in the pyriform sinuses, the valleculae, or the open airway. Where the bolus rests during the delay is a result of gravity, head posture, and the consistency of the food and is not the major symptom of a pharyngeal swallow delay. The critical symptom of delay is the location of the bolus head—in other words, whether it has progressed too far down into the pharynx before the pharyngeal swallow is activated. The bolus head must be differentiated from premature bolus loss. The bolus head is the leading edge of the main portion of the bolus. Premature bolus loss occurs during the oral preparatory or oral stages of the swallow as part of the bolus breaks away from the main portion of the bolus and falls over the tongue base. Premature bolus loss is not a delay in triggering the pharyngeal swallow.

If the bolus reaches the pyriform sinus, as shown in Figure 5.13, before the pharyngeal swallow is triggered, there is increased risk of aspiration as the pharyngeal swallow is activated, because the pyriform sinus is significantly shortened as the pharynx and larynx elevate during the pharyngeal swallow. If the pyriform sinuses fill with food or liquid during the delay in triggering the pharyngeal swallow, then when the pharynx and larynx are elevating, the contents of the pyriform sinuses are at high risk of being dumped into the airway, as shown in Figure 5.14. In patients with a delayed pharyngeal swallow in whom the bolus falls to the pyriform sinus, a chin-down posture may be less helpful (Shanahan et al., in press). The chin-down posture affects the P-A pharyngeal dimensions by narrowing the laryngeal entrance and the distance between the tongue base and pharyngeal wall. These changes occur above the level of the pyriform sinus. A chin-down posture does not change the degree of pharyngeal shortening that occurs during swallowing, nor does it prevent the contents of the pyriform sinus from emptying into the airway if the bolus reaches the pyriform sinus.

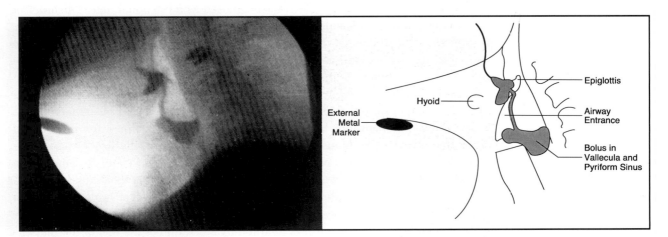

FIGURE 5.13.   A lateral videoprint and drawing of the oropharyngeal swallow showing the bolus in the pyriform sinus during the pharyngeal delay. Since the pharyngeal swallow has not been triggered, the airway is open, the pharyngeal walls are at rest, and the cricopharyngeal sphincter is closed. These events are initiated when the pharyngeal swallow is triggered. This patient is at greatest risk for aspiration when the pharyngeal swallow is finally triggered and the larynx and pharynx elevate as the initial events in the pharyngeal swallow. As the pharynx lifts, the pyriform sinuses are shortened and the food or liquid that has reached the pyriform sinuses during the delay is usually dumped into the airway, which is still open at this time.

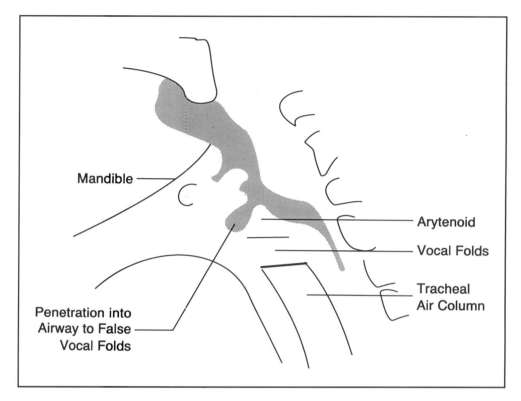

FIGURE 5.14.   A lateral drawing of the pharynx with bolus overflowing into the airway from the pyriform sinus as the pharyngeal swallow is triggered.

Occasionally the delayed pharyngeal swallow in which the bolus falls to the pyriform sinus during the delay has been misdiagnosed as a cricopharyngeal disorder or "late opening" of the cricopharyngeus. This is not a cricopharyngeal disorder, and the cricopharyngeal region is not dysfunctional. The sphincter is not opening because the "swallow center" or "central pattern generator" in the brain stem has not programmed it to open (i.e., the pharyngeal swallow has not been triggered).

Timing the pharyngeal delay.   In the report of the radiographic study, the duration of the pharyngeal delay should be included. This serves as a baseline measure against which treatment effects can be defined. The delay is timed from the initial video frame showing the bolus head passing the point where the lower edge of the mandible crosses the tongue base (as illustrated in Figures 5.11 and 5.12) until the first frame where the pharyngeal swallow is initiated (where laryngeal and hyoid elevation begin as a part of the pharyngeal swallow). In the pharyngeal swallow, elevation of the larynx and hyoid are the first events. These actions serve as a marker of triggering of the pharyngeal swallow, if it is followed by activation of the rest of the pharyngeal swallow. During a pharyngeal swallow delay, many patients struggle to stimulate a swallow, and in the struggle behavior, they move their tongue forward and backward and lift their larynx up and down, but these movements are not the same as those seen during the pharyngeal swallow. When timing the pharyngeal swallow delay, the movements of the larynx up and down as the tongue is moving to try to stimulate a swallow are not part of the pharyngeal swallow and should not be identified as such. It is easy to identify the triggering of the pharyngeal swallow by watching the swallow as it progresses and reversing the videotape in slow motion until the larynx first comes back to rest. Any laryngeal movements prior to the actual pharyngeal swallow should be considered part of the delay.

In normal young adult subjects, pharyngeal delay is minimal (0 to 0.2 sec). In normal subjects over age 60, there is a statistically significant prolongation of the pharyngeal delay to 0.5 sec (Tracy et al., 1989). We consider a delay of more than 1 sec, or an even shorter delay during which aspiration occurs, an abnormal delay in adults, regardless of age.

The pharyngeal triggering and delay time in infants and young children is quite different from that of adults because the bolus is collected in the valleculae before the pharyngeal swallow is triggered. In an infant, an abnormal delay is defined as more than 1 sec between the last tongue pump and the onset of the pharyngeal swallow, or aspiration occurring during bolus collection.

Disorders in the Pharyngeal Stage of Deglutition

The pharyngeal phase of deglutition begins when the pharyngeal swallow is triggered as the bolus passes the anterior faucial arch or back-base of the tongue and continues until the bolus passes through the cricopharyngeal region, or UES, or the pharyngoesophageal segment. Normal PTT is a maximum of 1 sec regardless of the patient's age or the material swallowed. For small-volume swallows, PTT is approximately 0.32 sec and increases as volume increases. Disorders of the pharyngeal phase of the swallow include dysfunctions of any of the neuromuscular components that actualize the pharyngeal swallow or characterize the pharyngeal response.

Nasal penetration during swallow—reduced velopharyngeal closure. When velopharyngeal closure is inadequate, material can backflow into the nose during swallowing, as shown in Figure 5.15. However, it is important to note that velopharyngeal

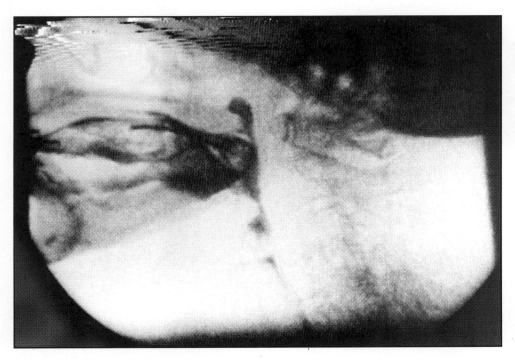

FIGURE 5.15.   A lateral view of the posterior oral cavity and pharynx illustrating nasal regurgitation of the bolus during the pharyngeal stage of swallow.

closure during the swallow lasts for only a fraction of a second as the bolus passes the velopharyngeal port. If nasal backflow occurs later in the swallow, it may be the result of a dysfunction farther down in the pharynx. If the bolus cannot pass through the pharynx into the esophagus, food, especially liquid, will often move back upward, and at that moment the velopharyngeal port is normally open, since velopharyngeal closure is complete only as the bolus passes the nasopharynx. When a patient complains of nasal leakage of food, a complete examination of the pharynx during swallow is warranted.

   Pseudoepiglottis (after total laryngectomy)—fold of mucosa at the base of the tongue.   After total laryngectomy some patients exhibit a fold of mucosa at the base of the tongue. This fold of tissue forms what appears to be an epiglottis when viewed radiographically in the lateral plane (see Figure 5.16). This pseudoepiglottis can look quite benign when viewed anatomically because it collapses against the base of the tongue and leaves an open pharynx posteriorly. However, when the patient attempts to swallow, whatever contraction occurs in the pharyngeal constrictors will pull the tissue fold posteriorly and narrow the pharynx so that the patient can barely move any food past the pseudoepiglottis. It is important to assess the effect of this tissue fold on swallow function physiologically through fluoroscopy, rather than depending solely on an anatomic examination.

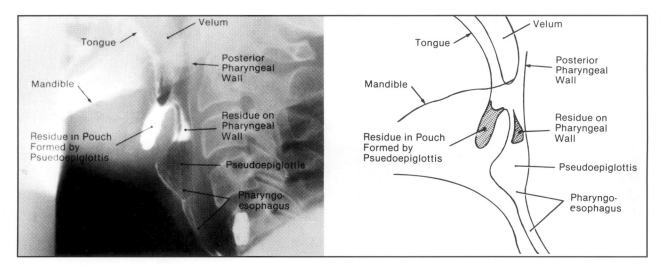

FIGURE 5.16.   A lateral radiographic view of the tongue base and pharynx in a total laryngectomee, illustrating a large pseudoepiglottis with residual food captured in the pouch created by the pseudoepiglottis. This patient is symptomatic for difficulty in swallowing.

Bony outgrowth from the cervical vertebrae—cervical osteophytes.   Bony outgrowths from the cervical vertebrae are known as cervical osteophytes (see Figure 5.17). At times they can be large enough to interfere with the swallow by narrowing the pharynx. At other times they may simply cause the patient to have the sensation of a swallowing disorder, that is, of "something there" when they swallow. During the radiographic study, the clinician should always scan the cervical vertebrae for any abnormalities.

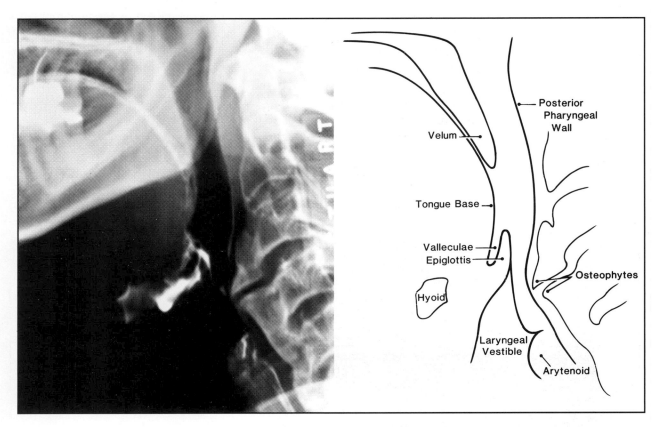

FIGURE 5.17.   A lateral radiographic view of the oral cavity and pharynx in a patient with large osteophytes on cervical vertebrae. Two of the vertebrae are also fused.

Coating on the pharyngeal walls after the swallow—reduced pharyngeal contraction bilaterally. After the swallow in normal individuals, there is only a minimal residue of material left in the pharynx. In many normal subjects there is no residue whatsoever. Older normal individuals do not exhibit any greater residue than younger adults. Figures 5.18 and 5.19 illustrate the range of normal pharyngeal residue. To some extent, the amount of coating in the pharynx will vary with the type of barium contrast given. Some types of barium will usually cause a greater amount of coating, even in normal individuals, than other types of barium. In general, if the pharyngeal structures are merely lightly coated with barium after the swallow, as if the barium has mixed with saliva or mucus, the amount of residue is normal. However, a significant amount of residual material on the pharyngeal walls, as judged by the apparent density of the material remaining, would be considered abnormal and a symptom of reduced pharyngeal contraction (peristalsis). A normal individual would dry swallow immediately after the food swallow to clear this residue. It is important, then, to watch for the patient's reaction to any residue left in the pharynx after the swallow. Whenever any larger amount of residue remains, the patient is at risk for aspiration following the swallow if he or she inhales any of the residue.

Vallecular residue—reduced posterior movement of the tongue base. When the bolus tail reaches the level of the tongue base and valleculae, the tongue base moves posteriorly to contact the anteriorly bulging pharyngeal wall. Approximately two-thirds of the distance between the tongue base and the pharyngeal wall at rest is encompassed by the posterior tongue-base movement and one third by the anterior movement of the pharyngeal wall (Kahrilas et al., 1991). Clearance of the valleculae appears to be the result of the tongue-base movement. When vallecular residue is noted, tongue base-movement should be observed to determine if it is adequate and

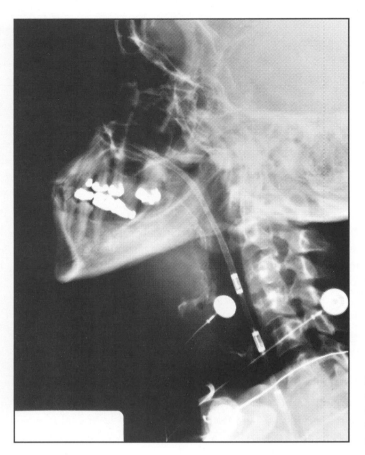

FIGURE 5.18. A lateral videoprint illustrating the oral cavity and pharynx after a normal swallow, showing no residue.

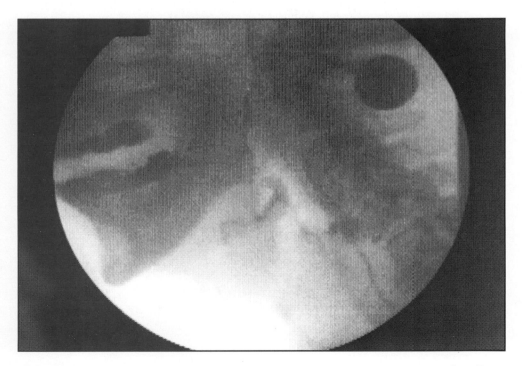

FIGURE 5.19. A lateral videoprint illustrating the oral cavity and pharynx after a normal swallow, showing the maximum residue observed in normal adult subjects of any age.

if it contacts the anteriorly bulging posterior pharyngeal wall. Figure 5.20 illustrates residue in the valleculae as the result of reduced posterior tongue-base motion. If the residue in the valleculae is substantial, the patient may be at risk of aspirating some or all of the residue during respiration after the swallow.

Coating in a depression on the pharyngeal wall—scar tissue; pharyngeal pouch. Collection of material in a depression on the pharyngeal wall may be an indication of the beginning of a pharyngeal pouch or scar tissue in the pharynx. If a patient has had a pharyngocutaneous fistula, the internal end of the fistula will often heal as a scar tissue depression, which will collect material during and after the swallow. As with any pharyngeal residue, the patient is at risk for aspiration after the swallow if a large amount of residue is present.

Residue at top of airway—reduced laryngeal elevation. In normal individuals, when the pharyngeal swallow is triggered, the larynx elevates to tuck itself under the base of the tongue, as a component of airway protection. During swallowing, the larynx elevates approximately 2 cm in normal adults (Jacob et al., 1989).

If laryngeal elevation during the swallow is mildly impaired, some residual material will remain on top of the larynx after the swallow. Pharyngeal contraction cannot completely clear material from the top of the airway when the larynx is in an abnormally lowered position. Thus, the patient is at risk for aspiration of the food sitting on top of the airway after the swallow when he or she opens the larynx to inhale following deglutition.

As the larynx elevates, the arytenoid cartilage is brought to a level where it is closer to the base of the epiglottis and can tilt forward to contact the base of the epiglottis and close the entrance to the airway. Moderately reduced laryngeal elevation can, therefore, result in inability of the arytenoid to tilt anteriorly enough to make good contact with the epiglottis, leaving the entrance to the airway slightly open and allowing penetration of the bolus into the airway entrance. If the larynx does not continue to lift to a normal degree and material has penetrated the airway entrance, it will remain in the airway entrance and be aspirated after the swallow. Some patients can compensate for reduced laryngeal elevation by tilting the arytenoid more anteriorly than normal; these patients will not have penetration into the airway entrance. Sometimes, these patients begin arytenoid tilting before the swallow begins, thus closing the airway entrance preventively before and during the swallow.

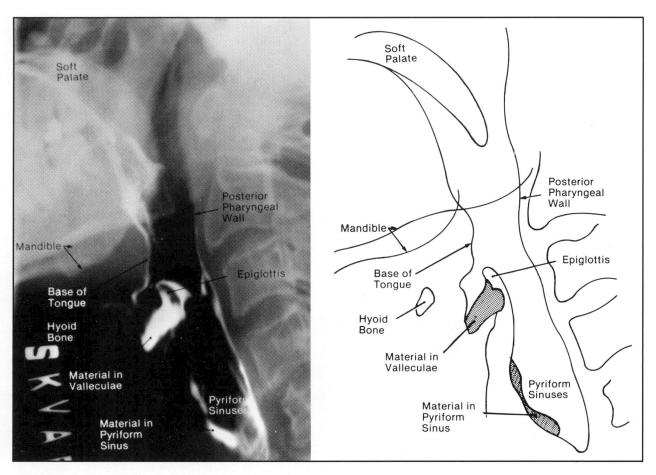

FIGURE 5.20.   A lateral videoprint illustrating residue in the valleculae as the result of reduced posterior tongue base-movement.

Laryngeal penetration and aspiration—reduced closure of the airway entrance (arytenoid to base of epiglottis). Laryngeal penetration occurs when food or liquid enters the vestibule or entrance of the airway to any extent down to the level of the true vocal folds. In contrast, aspiration involves entry of food into the airway below the vocal folds. Both penetration and aspiration are symptoms of a variety of swallowing problems. Observation of penetration or aspiration on an X-ray study of swallowing should cause the clinician to review the videotaped swallow carefully to identify the anatomic or physiologic cause of the penetration or aspiration.

Etiologies of laryngeal penetration. Laryngeal penetration can occur as a result of several etiologies. The bolus may penetrate to a variety of levels, as shown in Figures 5.21, 5.22, and 5.23. The bolus may enter the airway to the level of the middle of the arytenoid cartilage, the surface of the false vocal folds, or the true vocal folds. Penetration can occur if the larynx lifts inadequately and thus leaves the airway entrance slightly open, or if the arytenoid cartilage fails to tilt forward adequately to

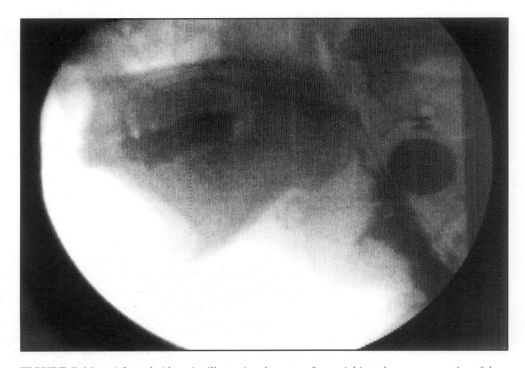

FIGURE 5.21. A lateral videoprint illustrating the entry of material into the topmost portion of the airway entrance because of a mild reduction in laryngeal elevation.

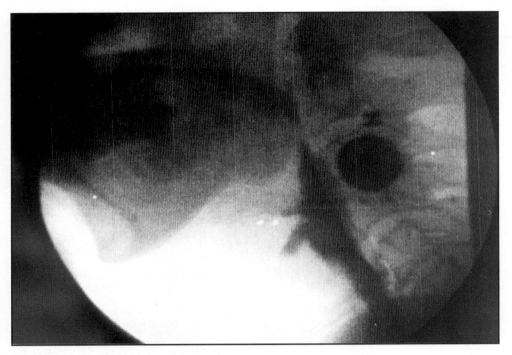

FIGURE 5.22. A lateral videoprint illustrating penetration of liquid into the airway entrance to the level of the false vocal folds because of moderately reduced laryngeal elevation.

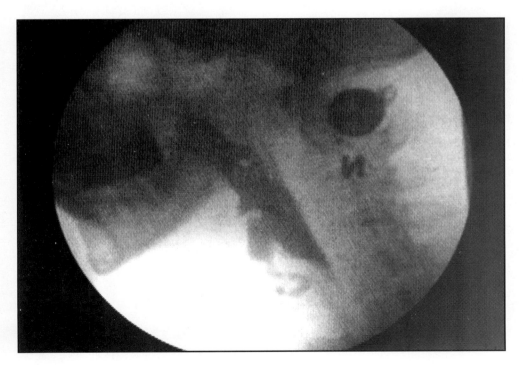

FIGURE 5.23. A lateral videoprint illustrating penetration of the bolus into the airway entrance to the level of the true vocal folds during a pharyngeal swallow delay, before the pharyngeal swallow was triggered. This 10-ml bolus has filled the pharynx and entered the laryngeal vestibule (airway entrance) to the surface of the true vocal folds.

close off the entrance to the airway. Penetration can also occur if the larynx lifts too slowly during the swallow; however, if the larynx lifts too slowly but eventually lifts to its full range of motion and closes, all of the penetrated material will be cleared from the airway entrance. Figures 5.24 and 5.25 illustrate penetration in supraglottic laryngectomees because of failure of the arytenoid to fully tilt and contact the retracting tongue base.

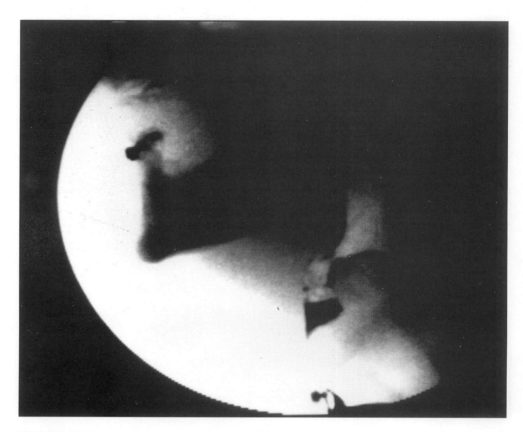

FIGURE 5.24. A supraglottic laryngectomee with material penetrating to the level of the surface of the true vocal folds.

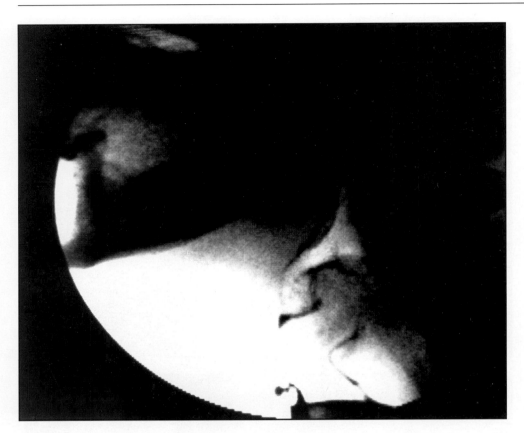

FIGURE 5.25.   A lateral radiographic view of a supraglottic laryngectomee with material on top of and under the vocal folds, indicating penetration with aspiration after the swallow.

In normal individuals, when laryngeal penetration occurs, the material in the airway is squeezed out during the swallow as the larynx continues to lift and close inferiorly to superiorly. Penetration is only a problem when the larynx fails to lift and close adequately during the course of the swallow and the penetrated material remains in the larynx afterward and is aspirated as the individual inhales following the swallow. Penetration may also occur if the bolus falls into the airway entrance before the pharyngeal swallow is triggered, that is, if penetration is due to a delay in triggering the pharyngeal swallow, as shown in Figure 5.23. If the patient who has a delayed pharyngeal swallow has the vocal folds closed during the delay, food or liquid may enter the airway entrance but may not proceed farther than the surface of the true vocal folds. When the pharyngeal swallow is triggered and the larynx lifts and closes from the level of the true vocal folds upward, this penetrated material is usually cleared efficiently from the airway, as shown in Figure 5.26.

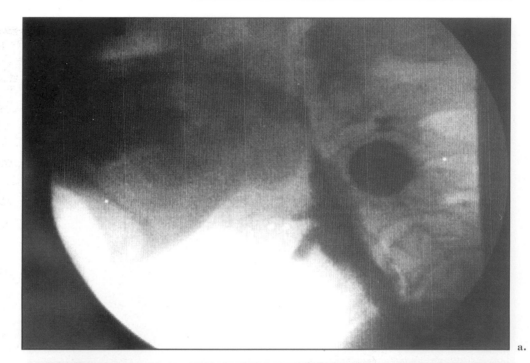

a.

b.

FIGURE 5.26.   Videoprints of lateral views of the pharynx showing the sequence of penetration of liquid into the larynx to the level of the false vocal folds during the swallow, and the clearance of this material as the swallow progresses. (*a*) The bolus has penetrated the laryngeal vestibule and is sitting on the false vocal folds. At this time, the pharyngeal swallow has triggered and the larynx and hyoid have just begun to lift and move forward. The cricopharyngeal region is not yet open. (*b*) Approximately 0.35 sec later, the hyoid and larynx have fully elevated and the penetrated liquid has been largely cleared from the larynx, squeezed upward by progressive laryngeal elevation and closure. There are very small remnants of liquid in the laryngeal vestibule, which may be aspirated after the swallow unless the patient coughs or clears the throat. The clearance mechanism for laryngeal penetration illustrated here occurs in normal subjects when occasional penetration into the laryngeal inlet occurs. The mechanism is highly successful in efficiently clearing the penetrated material, thereby eliminating risk of aspiration. If a patient's larynx does not elevate well after penetration has occurred, penetrated material will remain in the larynx until after the swallow, when it will be aspirated on the inhalation following the swallow.

Aspiration, like penetration, has a wide range of etiologies. When aspiration is seen on the videofluoroscopic study, the clinician should carefully review the video-taped swallow in slow motion and frame by frame to identify the etiology of the aspiration. Various etiologies are noted as each disorder is described in this book.

Aspiration during swallow—reduced laryngeal closure. During the pharyngeal phase of the swallow, the larynx closes at three levels or valves: (a) the true vocal folds, (b) the arytenoid to the base of the epiglottis, and (c) the aryepiglottic folds and epiglottis. If the larynx does not close adequately from bottom to top during the swallow, material will enter the airway during the swallow. It will appear as if the larynx is offering little or no obstruction to the flow of material into the airway, as shown in Figure 5.27 in a supraglottic laryngectomee.

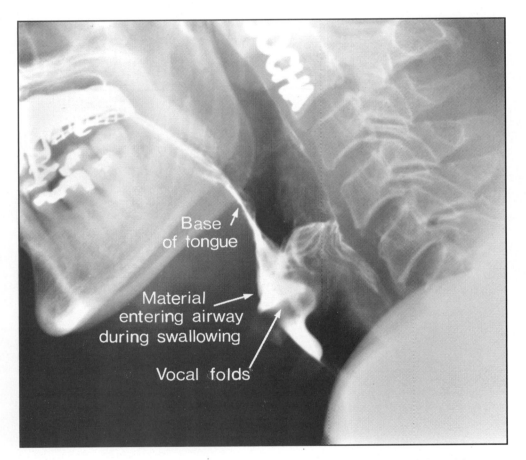

FIGURE 5.27.   A lateral radiographic view of a supraglottic laryngectomee with failure of the entrance to the airway (tongue base to arytenoid cartilage) and failure of the true vocal folds to close, with the bolus flowing through the airway into the trachea.

Stasis or residue in both pyriform sinuses—reduced anterior laryngeal movement; cricopharyngeal dysfunction; stricture.   Normally, little or no residual material is left in the pyriform sinuses after the swallow. When there is significant residue in both pyriform sinuses, it is a symptom of reduced anterior laryngeal movement and/or cricopharyngeal dysfunction (upper esophageal valve dysfunction) or stricture at the level of the opening of the esophagus. All other aspects of the swallow, including the triggering of the pharyngeal swallow, should be normal. If the pharyngeal swallow has not been triggered, a cricopharyngeal disorder cannot be diagnosed. Since anterior laryngeal movement controls cricopharyngeal opening and relaxation of the cricopharyngeal muscle is an enabling event, failure of this upper sphincter opening must be investigated further to determine which component is disordered. Usually, pharyngeal manometry must be combined with videofluoroscopy (described in Chapter 7) to assess these components. Figure 5.28 illustrates residue in the pyriform sinuses in a 3-year-old, head-injured child with a cricopharyngeal, reduced-anterior-laryngeal movement disorder.

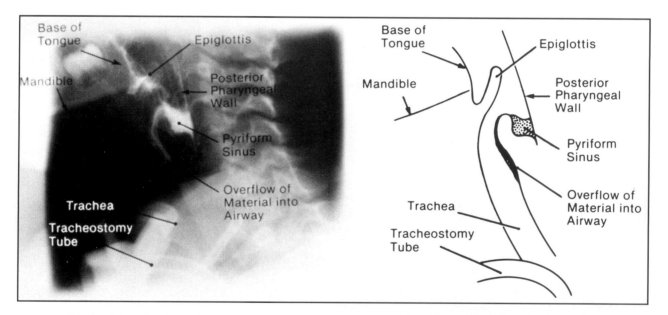

FIGURE 5.28.   A lateral radiographic view of the pharynx in a 3-year-old head-injured child illustrating residue in the pyriform sinus because of reduced laryngeal anterior motion and reduced cricopharyngeal opening, with aspiration of material over the arytenoid cartilage.

Residue throughout the pharynx—generalized reduction in pharyngeal pressure. If residue in the pyriform sinuses is combined with residue in other parts of the pharynx, such as the valleculae or the pharyngeal walls, as shown in Figure 5.29, it is a symptom of generalized dysfunction in pharyngeal pressure generation in the swallow, not an isolated cricopharyngeal problem. Generalized pharyngeal dysfunction includes reduced posterior movement of the tongue base and reduced pharyngeal wall movement. Often, laryngeal elevation is also reduced.

Pharyngeal transit time (in seconds). Normally, pharyngeal transit time is less than 1 sec regardless of the patient's age or the consistency of the food. Slowed PTT must be considered in combination with OTT to determine the full duration of the oropharyngeal swallow. The speed of the swallow through the oral and pharyngeal stages is one important factor in determining whether a patient is going to get sufficient nutrition by mouth, as discussed later in Chapter 8.

Other. This space is provided for the clinician to note any other abnormal movement patterns or structural problems that may be observed during the pharyngeal phase of deglutition in the lateral plane. An example of this would be a pharyngeal pouch.

Posture or treatment introduced. Space is provided to note any treatment procedures introduced and evaluated during the radiographic study.

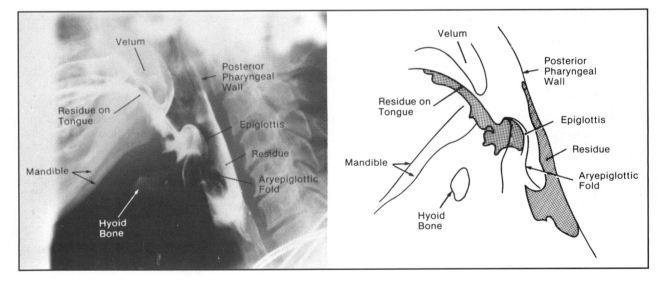

FIGURE 5.29. A lateral radiographic view of the oral cavity and pharynx in a patient with generalized reduction in pharyngeal contraction and tongue-base posterior motion, with residual food coating the posterior pharyngeal walls, tongue base, valleculae, and pyriform sinuses.

Disorders in the Cervical Esophageal Aspect of Deglutition

The cervical esophageal aspect of deglutition involves the initial peristaltic wave in the esophageal musculature. While the patient is being viewed radiographically in the lateral plane during the MBS, the cervical esophageal aspect of deglutition will be observable. If there is any question about the patient's esophageal function, an esophageal study (traditional barium swallow) should be performed after the modified barium swallow is completed, or the patient should be referred to a gastroenterologist for assessment. In this way the patient's ability to swallow without aspiration will have been established and the barium swallow can be done safely. If the patient cannot swallow safely without aspiration, the esophageal examination can be postponed until the risk of aspiration is eliminated.

The esophageal stage of deglutition cannot be modified by therapy, though postural changes are sometimes helpful. It is, however, important that the swallowing clinician be aware of the esophageal disorders that can masquerade as pharyngeal-phase swallowing disorders because they can cause backflow of the material out of the esophagus into the pharynx, thus also causing aspiration. A number of these disorders will be defined here, particularly those that may present a diagnostic problem for the swallowing therapist and radiologist performing MBS procedures.

Esophageal-to-pharyngeal backflow—esophageal abnormality.   Esophageal-to-pharyngeal backflow may occur because of a number of esophageal disorders. Backflow of material out of the esophagus into the pharynx requires the upper esophageal sphincter to open. Once material has come out of the esophagus into the pharynx, it may overflow into the airway, causing aspiration and possibly symptoms of a pharyngeal swallowing disorder. Patients with esophageal backflow may exhibit redness in the arytenoid area of the larynx on indirect laryngoscopy if the material overflowing into the airway contains stomach acid. They may also complain of a burning sensation in their pharynx and esophagus, or frequent gagging or coughing. Aspirated material that contains any gastric acid is more irritating to the lungs than aspirated saliva or food.

Tracheoesophageal (TE) fistula.   Occasionally, a fistula (hole) can develop in the soft tissue common wall between the trachea and the esophagus. This fistula tract allows food entering the esophagus to flow back into the trachea. Patients with TE fistulae have symptoms similar to those of patients who aspirate after the swallow for other reasons, such as coughing after the swallow. Thus, they may be referred to a swallowing therapist for evaluation. Any time a patient with a history of possible aspiration is referred for a radiographic study and the MBS results are normal, the radiographic study should be continued and the esophagus evaluated carefully to determine the presence or absence of a TE fistula. Since the fistula is usually located at T1–T3, the shoulders often shadow the radiographic image in the lateral plane. To improve visualization of this part of the esophagus and trachea, the patient's shoulders should be turned diagonally while the patient's head and body remain in the lateral view. Swallows should be repeated with the patient in this position and the fluoroscopic tube lowered to the base of the cervical esophagus in order to visualize the fistula tract.

Zenker's diverticulum. A diverticulum is a side pocket that forms when pharyngeal or esophageal muscle herniates. A Zenker's diverticulum occurs in the area immediately above or below the cricopharyngeal region (upper esophageal sphincter). One theory of its genesis states that a hypertonic cricopharyngeus muscle requires the patient to increase pharyngeal pressures to push food through the upper esophageal sphincter, thus causing the esophageal tissue to herniate. On X ray, the diverticulum appears as a round balloon that fills with radiopaque material as the patient swallows.

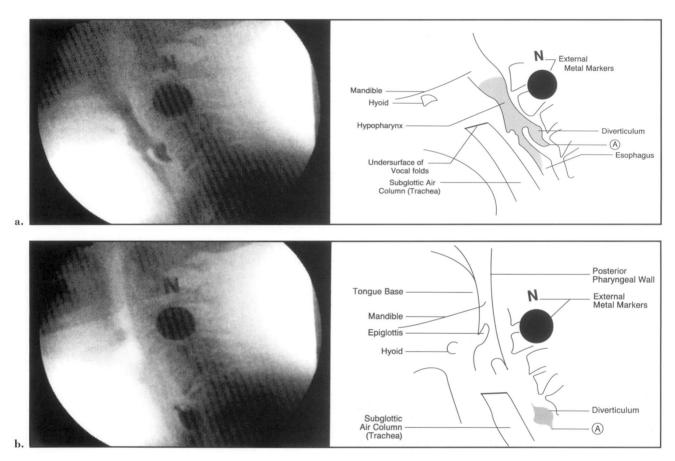

FIGURE 5.30. The dynamics of filling and backflow into the pharynx from a Zenker's diverticulum. (*a*) A lateral videoprint and drawing of the pharyngeal and early cervical esophageal aspect of swallow, with the hyoid and airway well elevated, the cricopharyngeal region open, and the bolus flowing into the diverticulum and the cricopharyngeal region. As a part of the pharyngeal wall, the diverticulum lifts with the larynx and pharynx during swallow. Point *A* is the inferior aspect of the diverticulum. (*b*) The pharynx and cervical esophagus at rest, with the airway open, the cricopharyngeal region closed, and the diverticulum filled with residual barium. Note that the base of the diverticulum (point *A*) lowers two vertebral bodies from its elevated position during swallow (shown in *a*) to its rest position.

After the swallow, the diverticulum usually empties of material. Upon emptying, this material may fall into the airway, causing aspiration after the swallow. Figure 5.30 presents a Zenker's diverticulum and the dynamics of the fistula causing backflow.

Reflux.   The term *reflux* indicates a specific type of backflow: backflow of food from the stomach to the esophagus. In the MBS, reflux is usually not diagnosed because the study is not viewing the *lower* esophageal sphincter. If reflux is suspected from the patient's history, consultation with a gastroenterologist is indicated.

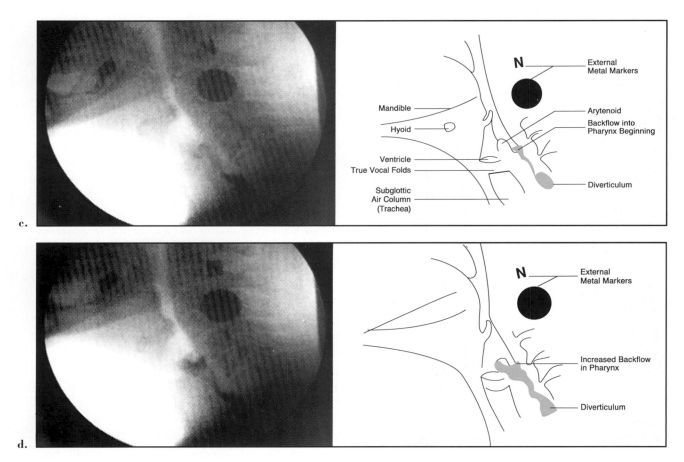

Figure 5.30 (continued). (*c*) Residual contents of the diverticulum beginning to flow back upward into the pharynx. (*d*) Increase in backflow, causing a larger amount of food to reenter the pharynx (pyriform sinus).

The Posterior-Anterior View

The P-A radiographic view allows the clinician to examine the symmetry of structures and function in the oral cavity and pharynx during deglutition and in the larynx during phonation. In approximately 80% of normal individuals, the bolus divides fairly equally to pass down the two sides of the pharynx and into the esophagus. The other 20% swallow unilaterally (Logemann, Kahrilas, Kobara, & Vakil, 1989). The P-A plane also allows assessment of oral functions during mastication and preparation to swallow.

Oral Preparatory Phase

During the oral preparatory phase in the P-A view, the clinician can examine (a) the ability of the tongue to lateralize material and (b) the pattern of jaw motion in crushing the food during mastication. The shape of the tongue in holding the bolus prior to.initiation of the swallow in the oral cavity can also be assessed. The sides of the tongue should be in contact with the lateral alveolus with a central groove down the midline surrounding the bolus. Disorders in these functions are described here.

Unable to align teeth—reduced mandibular movement. Some patients, particularly those who have had surgery to the lower jaw, will have difficulty putting the mandible into proper occlusion for chewing. This is an indication of reduced mandibular range of motion; it usually occurs when part of the mandible has been removed.

Unable to lateralize material with the tongue—reduced tongue lateralization. During chewing, the tongue lateralizes food, moving it to the side of the oral cavity, placing it onto the teeth. An inability by the patient to lateralize food from the midline is an indication of reduced tongue movement laterally.

Unable to mash materials—reduced tongue elevation. If a patient cannot lateralize food to the teeth for chewing, he or she may compensate or be asked to compensate by vertically crushing the food between the tongue and palate. An inability by the patient to accomplish this mashing of food is an indication of reduced tongue elevation to the hard palate.

Material falls into the lateral sulcus—reduced buccal muscle tension or tone. If, as the patient is chewing, material falls into the lateral sulcus, it is an indication of reduced facial-buccal muscle tension or tone. It is facial-buccal muscle tension that closes the lateral sulcus and throws food medially to the tongue during mastication.

Material. falls to the floor of the mouth—reduced tongue control. Food falling onto the floor of the mouth as the patient is chewing is a symptom of reduced tongue control.

Bolus spread across the mouth—reduced lingual shaping and fine tongue control. When a liquid or paste bolus is placed into the oral cavity, the tongue normally shapes around the bolus to hold it in a cohesive ball. Also, after chewing, the tongue normally pulls the food together into a single bolus and shapes itself around the bolus so that the sides of the tongue are sealed to the superior lateral alveolar ridge. If the patient is unable to shape his or her tongue around the bolus (i.e., to elevate one or both sides of the tongue or form a central groove to contain the food), it is an indication of reduced fine control of the tongue.

Posture or treatment introduced. This space allows notation of postures or other treatment strategies introduced in the radiographic study and their effects.

Pharyngeal Phase of Deglutition

The pharyngeal stage of the swallow, as assessed in the P-A view, provides information on the unilateral nature of any pharyngeal swallowing disorder.

Unilateral vallecular residue—unilateral damage to posterior movement of the tongue base. Food left in the valleculae on only one side after the swallow indicates dysfunction of one side of the tongue base or the pharyngeal constrictors. This residue, if it is a large amount, may be aspirated after the swallow.

Residue in one pyriform sinus—unilateral pharyngeal wall damage. Residue in only one pyriform sinus indicates unilateral dysfunction of the pharyngeal walls. This may result from neurologic or structural damage. Whenever there is a large amount of residue remaining in the pharynx after the swallow, the patient is at risk for aspiration after the swallow if any of the residue is inhaled or falls into the airway. Figures 5.31 and 5.32 illustrate unilateral pharyngeal wall damage in an adult and a child.

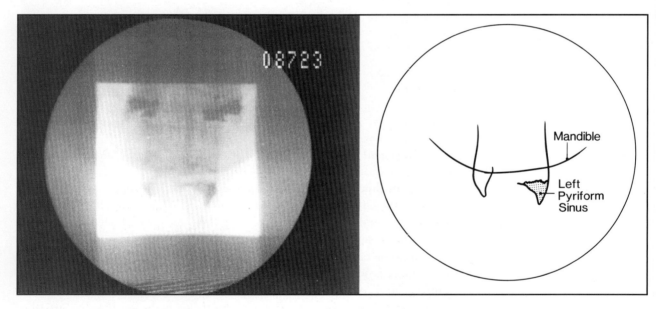

FIGURE 5.31. A posterior-anterior view of the oral cavity and pharynx in a brain-stem stroke patient with unilateral pharyngeal-wall weakness causing food residue in the impaired side of the pharynx. The apex or tip of the pyriform sinus is lower on the impaired side.

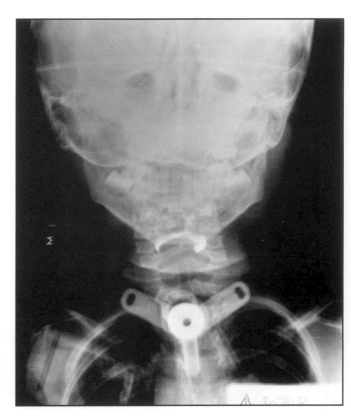

FIGURE 5.32.   A posterior-anterior view of a 2-year-old child with unilateral pharyngeal-wall weakness as a result of Wardnig-Hoffman disease. There is increased residue on the left side of the child's pharynx. A tracheostomy tube is also in place.

Reduced laryngeal movement medially—reduced vocal fold adduction. With the patient's head tilted backward to get the mandible out of view, vocal fold adduction can be evaluated. The patient should be asked to repeat "ah, ah, ah" rapidly to facilitate the clinician's localization of the vocal folds. When the vocal folds are identified, the patient should inhale, prolong "ah" for several seconds, inhale, then prolong "ah" for several seconds. This will reveal vocal fold abduction and adduction and allow the clinician to assess the symmetry of vocal fold movement, particularly on adduction. Whenever there is reduced movement of one vocal fold, it indicates reduced laryngeal adduction and a possible unilateral adductor vocal fold paresis or paralysis. This may be a cause of aspiration during the swallow because the larynx may be unable to protect the airway during the pharyngeal swallow.

Unequal height of the vocal folds. Occasionally, in partially laryngectomized patients, the reconstructed larynx on one side may be at a different vertical position than the vocal fold on the unoperated side. Thus, when the patient attempts to close the larynx to protect the airway during the swallow, even if both sides of the larynx move well, the two sides of the larynx do not meet each other and airway closure is incomplete, as shown in Figure 5.33. This is another cause of aspiration during the swallow, because the larynx is not closed sufficiently to protect the airway.

Other. On the fluoroscopy examination form, there is room for the clinician to note problems that are observed other than those listed. The clinician can note, therefore, any other abnormal radiographic symptoms that may be observed during the MBS but that may not be listed on the videofluorographic worksheet.

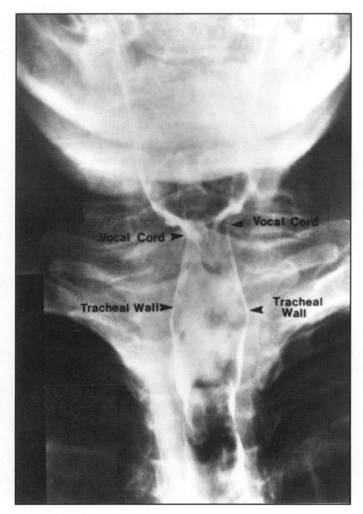

FIGURE 5.33. Anterior view of the larynx illustrating unequal height of the vocal folds.

NOTES

N O T E S

CHAPTER 6

Measurements of Swallow from Videofluorographic Studies

I
n the last five years, a number of clinical investigators have begun to use measurements of particular aspects of oropharyngeal swallowing to better describe and define the nature of swallowing disorders and to compare swallow measures in patients with various disorders to normal swallowing measures (Dantas et al., 1989; Dantas et al., 1990; Jacob et al., 1989; Kahrilas et al., 1992; Logemann, Kahrilas, Kobara, & Vakil, 1989; Logemann et al., 1992). This chapter will describe these measurements and how they can be made from videofluorographic studies. Currently, many of these measures are not routinely used clinically. However, many of them have clinical application to the assessment of a patient's progress in therapy.

To facilitate measurements from videofluorographic studies, the videotape should be recorded with timing information on each video frame or field. Some VCRs are capable of automatically recording timing information on each field (60 fields/sec) or frame (30 frames/sec) of the videotape. For recorders that do not have this capability, a countertimer can be interfaced between the incoming video signal from the fluoroscopic monitor and the VCR. The counter timer can be set to record 100th-of-a-second intervals or consecutive numbers on each field or frame on the videotape. Since videotape contains 30 frames/sec, or 60 fields/sec (two fields are used to define a frame), if the timer runs at 100th of a second, there will be more numbers than there are frames or fields, and some numbers will be skipped. If the timer runs at 60 fields/sec, each field will be numbered consecutively with no missing numbers. Timing information on each video frame facilitates the observer's identification of specific points on the videotape and serves as a reference for a return to those frames at a later time.

Currently, measurements of swallowing include (a) temporal measures of bolus movement, (b) oropharyngeal swallow efficiency, (c) temporal measures of specific events within the swallow and their coordination, (d) coordination of pharyngeal swallow events, (e) distance measures of structural movements, and (f) biomechanical measures of structural movement patterns over time from the onset of the swallow. Each of these measures provides different kinds of information and will be described separately.

Duration of Bolus Movement

Measures of the duration of bolus movement include oral transit time (OTT), pharyngeal transit time (PTT), pharyngeal delay time (PDT), and esophageal transit time (ETT).

Oral Transit Time

This is defined as the length of time it takes the bolus to move through the oral cavity from the first frame showing backward movement of food until the bolus head (leading edge) or tail passes a landmark in the posterior oral cavity, defined variously as the anterior faucial arch, the back of the tongue, or the spot where the lower edge of the ramus of the mandible crosses the tongue base. Investigators have used various landmarks to determine the beginning and end of oral transit (Sonies, Parent, Morrish, & Baum, 1988; Tracy et al., 1989). If bolus head movement is used to define the onset and termination of OTT, then OTT will shorten as bolus volume increases because the bolus head is located more posteriorly in the mouth as bolus size increases. If bolus tail movement is used to define the onset and termination of OTT, OTT will be relatively constant across volumes. Generally, when the bolus head reaches the point where the shadow of the ramus of the mandible crosses the tongue base, as shown in Figure 6.1, the pharyngeal stage of swallow should be activated. OTTs have been found to lengthen slightly with age and bolus consistency (thicker boluses result in slightly slower OTTs). OTT is always under 1.5 sec in normal subjects and is usually less than 1 sec.

Pharyngeal Transit Time

This is defined as the time it takes the bolus to move through the pharynx from the point at which the bolus head passes the back of the tongue or the ramus of the

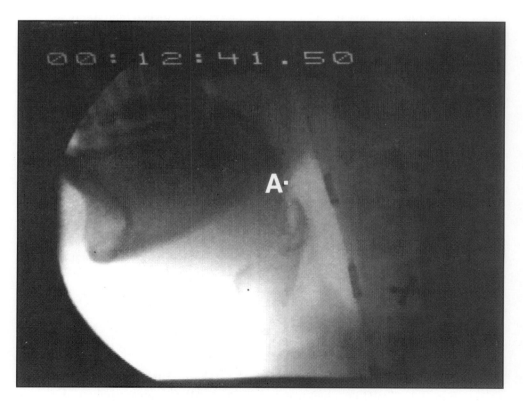

FIGURE 6.1.   A lateral videoprint with the point (*A*) identifying where the lower edge of the ramus of the mandible crosses the tongue base.

mandible until the bolus tail passes through the cricopharyngeal region, which is located behind the cricoid cartilage, approximately 1 cm below the true vocal folds (Kahrilas et al., 1988).

Pharyngeal Delay Time

PDT is a component of PTT. It is defined as the time from the bolus head arrival at the point where the shadow of the lower edge of the mandible crosses the tongue base until the pharyngeal swallow is triggered. Triggering or onset of the pharyngeal swallow is defined as the first video frame showing laryngeal elevation as a part of the pharyngeal swallowing complex. Pharyngeal delay increases significantly with age but not with bolus volume: under age 60, delay is an average of 0.24 sec; over age 60, mean delay is 0.36 sec (Tracy et al., 1989).

Esophageal Transit Time

ETT is measured as the time it takes the bolus to move through the esophagus from the time the bolus head enters the esophagus at the cricopharyngeal region until the tail of the bolus enters the stomach at the lower esophageal sphincter.

Normative values for each of these measurements vary somewhat from study to study, but in general they are thought to be approximately 1 sec for OTT, 0.3 to 1 sec for PTT, and 8 to 20 sec for ETT. Transit times do vary systematically in most individuals with the characteristics of the bolus. To date, transit times have been found to vary with bolus volume and bolus consistency. The effects of other bolus variables have not been studied at this time.

Oropharyngeal Swallow Efficiency (OPSE)

Recently, we have used another summary measure, OPSE, to define overall swallow function (Logemann & Kahrilas, 1990; Logemann, Kahrilas, Kobara, & Vakil, 1989). To calculate OPSE, the clinician reexamines the tape and approximates the percentage of the bolus swallowed into the esophagus (not including residue in the mouth or pharynx or any food that is aspirated) on the first swallow of each bolus. If a patient uses three swallows to clear a bolus, only the first is measured. Then oral and pharyngeal transit times are calculated for the first swallow of the bolus. Thus, the formula for calculating OPSE is: percentage of the bolus swallowed into the esophagus divided by oral plus pharyngeal transit times.

Since normal subjects swallow approximately 100% of the bolus in approximately 1.8 sec, normal oropharyngeal swallow efficiency is 40 or above. If OTT is faster, then OPSE increases. If a dysphagia is present, it will cause residue that reduces the percentage swallowed, create aspiration that reduces the amount swallowed, or slow transit times. In all of these examples, OPSE is reduced. OPSE is meant to represent a *global* measure of swallow function, taking into account all the aspects or effects of dysphagia (i.e., slow swallow, inefficient swallow leaving residue, and unsafe swallow resulting in aspiration); it can be used to track a patient's swallowing recovery over time and represent that recovery numerically. All of these measures of bolus movement can be made by observing the videotaped swallow in slow motion and frame by frame.

Temporal Measures of Swallow Events

Temporal measures of swallow events include the duration of velopharyngeal closure, laryngeal closure, and cricopharyngeal opening. These measures are defined as follows:

- *Duration of velopharyngeal closure:* The number of video frames exhibiting contact of the velum to the posterior pharyngeal wall multiplied by 0.033 sec (the duration of one video frame)
- *Duration of airway closure:* The number of video frames exhibiting contact of the arytenoid to the base of the epiglottis or absence of air in the laryngeal entrance multiplied by 0.033 sec (the duration of one video frame)
- *Duration of cricopharyngeal opening:* The number of video frames exhibiting a space (opening) between the anterior and posterior walls of the cricopharyngeal region multiplied by 0.033 sec (the duration of one video frame)

Completing these temporal measures on a patient's swallows enables the clinician to compare the function of specific aspects of the patient's pharyngeal swallow with normal swallows. Currently, there are only a few studies providing normative values for these measures, so their clinical usefulness is not yet widespread (Cook, Dodds, Dantas, Kern, et al., 1989; Cook, Dodds, Dantas, Massey, et al., 1989; Dantas et al., 1990; Jacob et al., 1989; Kahrilas et al., 1988; Kahrilas et al., 1992; Kahrilas et al., in press; Logemann et al., 1992). However, it is likely that in the next few years, increasing numbers of studies will use these measures to define oropharyngeal swallowing physiology, and a larger normative data base by age group will be available for clinical reference. These measures also enable the clinician to determine whether the patient's swallow produces the same systematic changes with increasing bolus volume as normal swallow does. For example, in normal subjects, the duration of cricopharyngeal opening and the duration of airway closure increase systematically as the bolus volume increases. Cricopharyngeal opening duration for liquid swallows increases from 0.36 sec at 1 ml to 0.42 sec at 5 ml, 0.56 sec at 10 ml, and 0.64 sec at 20 ml (Jacob et al., 1989; Tracy et al., 1989). Airway closure duration increases from 0.48 sec on 1-ml liquid swallow to 0.5 sec on 5-ml swallows, 0.61 sec on 10-ml swallows, and 0.58 sec on 20-ml swallows (Logemann et al., 1992). Providing successively larger measured volumes to a dysphagic patient, as tolerated, enables the clinician to examine the compliance of the patient's swallow to increasing bolus volume as compared to normal subjects. Obviously, some dysphagic patients cannot safely handle large (5-ml, 10-ml, or 20-ml) volumes. If a patient swallows a large bolus in three or four segments rather than as a whole, or if the patient cannot maintain lip closure to keep the measured bolus in the mouth, these measures cannot be made.

Coordination of Pharyngeal Swallow Events

To measure the coordination of pharyngeal swallow events, one event must be selected as time 0. The event most commonly used is the first video frame showing cricopharyngeal opening. With this video frame as time 0, the onset and termination of all other oropharyngeal swallow events can be measured in relation to it. All events that begin before time 0 are indicated as negative values, and all events occurring after time 0 are noted as positive values. A time line, such as the one for a normal subject illustrated in Figure 6.2, can be generated for each of the patient's swallows and compared to the normal pattern of pharyngeal swallow coordination for that swallow volume.

Range of Structural Movement

To measure the extent of movement of oral or pharyngeal structures during a swallow, a "ruler" must be placed in the radiographic field during the videofluoroscopic study to account for magnification. A coin of known diameter such as a dime, taped at the midline under the patient's chin, can serve as the ruler. When measuring the distance an oropharyngeal structure moves during the swallow, the clinician should note where the structure was located on a video frame held in pause mode at the onset of the swallow and trace the outline of the structure, the coin, and several cervical vertebrae from that video frame onto tracing paper. Then, observing the structure's movement throughout the swallow, the clinician can select the video frame showing maximal movement of the structure, frame-pause that point, and retrace the same structures traced on the first selected frame. Finally, the distance moved by the structure of

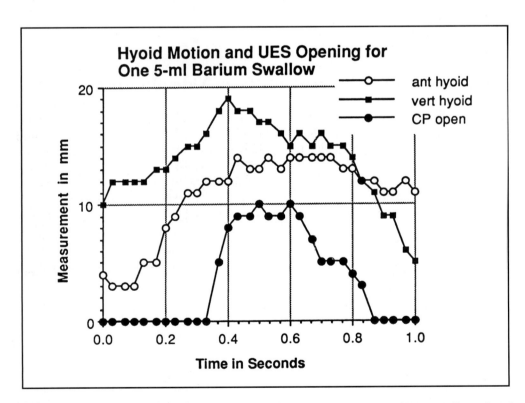

FIGURE 6.2. Plots of hyoid motion and cricopharyngeal opening over time during a single 5-ml swallow of barium liquid. Multiple plots of structural movement enable assessment of coordination of pharyngeal structures during swallow. Time 0 is the onset of vertical hyoid movement.

interest can be calculated by measuring the absolute distance from baseline to maximal movement and multiplying by the magnification correction factor derived from the coin. For example, if the maximum diameter of the coin is actually 1 cm, but on the X-ray tracing its maximum diameter is 2 cm, then the distance moved by the target structure measured on the tracing paper should be divided by 2, thus correcting for magnification created by the fluoroscopy.

Biomechanical Analysis

The sixth type of measurement, biomechanical analysis, involves tracking the movement of specific oropharyngeal structures over time from the onset to the termination of the swallow (Logemann, Kahrilas, Begelman, Dodds, & Pauloski, 1989). These types of measurements are most easily made by computer. Video frames containing the swallows of interest are digitized, recalled from computer memory one by one, and marked for the location of each structure of interest. In addition to marking the structures of interest, such as the hyoid bone or the larynx, a reference point (a point that does not move during deglutition), a reference distance to account for magnification, and the postural angle are also marked for each video frame. The computer then stores the coordinate locations of each structure on each frame by measuring them against the reference point, such as the sixth cervical vertebra, and correcting for the reference distance and postural angle. Graphs of distance over time are then generated for the structures of interest throughout the swallow, as shown in Figure 6.3. Such plots have been used to improve our understanding of cricopharyngeal opening, airway closure, and tongue-base and pharyngeal-wall movement (Dodds et al., 1989; Jacob et al., 1989; Kahrilas et al., in press; Logemann et al., 1992).

Applications of Measurements from Videofluoroscopy

Currently, the various measurements of oropharyngeal swallow described above are not widely used in clinical assessment of dysphagia, except for oral, pharyngeal, and esophageal transit times and pharyngeal delay time. However, over the next 5 to 6 years, it may become evident that selected measurements of particular aspects of the oral or pharyngeal stages of swallow are important in identifying particular disorders or in quantifying the effects of treatment strategies. For example, temporal measurements of selected events in the pharyngeal swallow can be used to describe the functioning of various valves in the oropharyngeal region. Durations of velopharyngeal closure, laryngeal closure, and cricopharyngeal opening have received the greatest attention, since each represents a critical valve along the pathway of bolus movement from the mouth to the esophagus. Measures of the duration of airway closure or cricopharyngeal opening may be used as indicators of treatment efficacy if therapy is directed at improving airway closure or cricopharyngeal opening. Table 6.1 outlines the applicability of various measures as treatment efficacy data for particular treatment strategies.

It is important for clinicians to continually review the dysphagia literature to determine those measurements that may be helpful in clinical evaluation of dysphagic patients. There may come a time when such measurements become a standard part of the evaluation of swallowing in at least selected types of dysphagic patients.

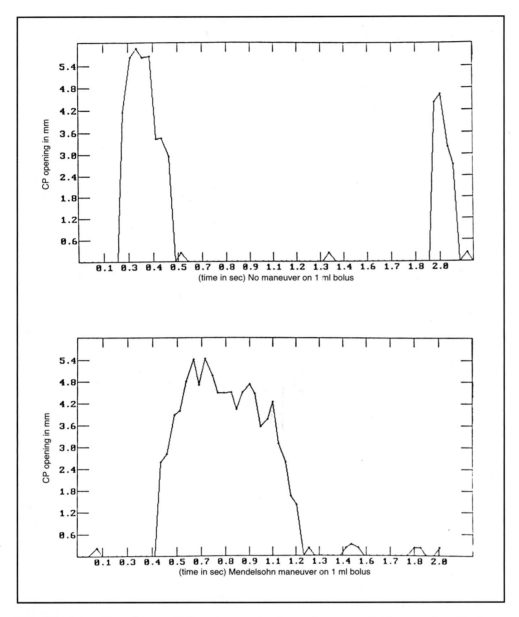

FIGURE 6.3.   Plots of laryngeal elevation over time in a patient accomplishing normal swallowing and the Mendelsohn maneuver, illustrating the ability of biomechanical analysis to plot the position of the larynx during a normal swallow and during therapeutic strategies.

TABLE 6.1 Measures of Swallowing That Are Useful in Determining the Efficacy of Treatment During the Radiographic Study of Oropharyngeal Swallow

MEASURES	TREATMENT EFFICACY APPLICATION

Oral transit time	Exercises to improve oral control
	    Tongue range of motion
	    Tongue coordination

Pharyngeal delay time	Therapy to improve triggering of the pharyngeal swallow Thermal and tactile stimulation; suck swallow
Duration of velopharyngeal closure	Techniques to improve velopharyngeal closure
Duration of airway closure at entrance	Supersupraglottic swallow; effortful breath hold and adduction exercises
Duration of cricopharyngeal opening	Mendelsohn maneuver
Coordination of pharyngeal swallow events	Mendelsohn maneuver
Extent of laryngeal elevation	Mendelsohn maneuver; falsetto
Extent of anterior hyoid motion	Mendelsohn maneuver
Extent of vertical hyoid motion	Mendelsohn maneuver, falsetto
Extent of tongue base motion to pharyngeal wall	Effortful swallow; tongue-base retraction exercises
Oropharyngeal swallow efficiency	Any therapy to improve swallowing function (compensatory or direct)

NOTES

Attaining Proficiency in Measurement and Observation from Radiographic Studies

As in most skills, interpretation and measurement of radiographic studies require practice. Each member of a clinical staff responsible for interpreting videofluoroscopic studies of oropharyngeal swallow should practice until a level of "acceptable proficiency" is reached. Acceptable proficiency levels must be established by each facility. In our clinical swallowing laboratory, clinicians must be able to make the observations listed in Table 6.2 with no greater difference between their own repeated judgments (intraobserver reliability) and between their judgments and those of other experienced clinicians on the staff (interobserver reliability) than is shown in Table 6.2 before they are allowed to interpret videofluoroscopic studies independently. A number of training videotapes are available to assist clinicians in learning to make these observations. A listing of available tapes and their suppliers is included in Appendix C.

TABLE 6.2   Target Levels of Reliability from Temporal Analysis, in Seconds (greatest difference acceptable on repeated measures by the same observer [intraobserver] and by two observers [interobserver])

MEASURE	INTEROBSERVER RELIABILITY	INTRAOBSERVER RELIABILITY
Oral transit time	.21	.10
Pharyngeal transit time	.15	.15
Duration of velopharyngeal closure	.06	.06
Duration of laryngeal closure	.06	.06
Duration of cricopharyngeal opening	.06	.06
Duration of hyoid movement	.33	.33
Duration of laryngeal elevation	.33	33
Onset of oral transit	.15	.15
Bolus head reaches point where mandible crosses tongue base	.03	.03
Bolus over base of tongue	.09	.09
Start of soft palate elevation	.12	.12
First soft palate contact to posterior pharyngeal wall	.06	.06
Greatest soft palate elevation	.18	.18
Last soft palate contact to posterior pharyngeal wall	.06	.06
Onset of hyoid movement	.21	.21
Maximum hyoid movement	.12	.12
Hyoid return to rest	.21	.21
Onset of laryngeal elevation	.21	.21
First maximum laryngeal elevation	.12	.12
Last maximum laryngeal elevation	.12	.12
Laryngeal return to rest	.21	.21
First laryngeal closure	.06	.06
Last laryngeal closure	.06	.06
First cricopharyngeal opening	.06	.06
Last cricopharyngeal opening	.06	.06

Combining Videofluorographic Studies with Other Methodologies for Studying Swallow

In the last several years, several investigators have combined videofluorographic studies of oropharyngeal swallow with other methodologies for assessing swallowing physiology in order to increase the amount of information that can be gathered about normal and abnormal swallowing function. Two techniques have most frequently been used in combination with videofluorography: manometry and surface electromyography.

Manometry and Videofluorography

Until recently, manometric studies of the pharynx were used only to study the upper esophageal sphincter. Manometry is difficult to interpret in the pharynx because positioning of the sensors cannot be identified accurately or easily without X-ray visualization. Combining manometry, which measures pressures in the pharynx and the upper esophageal sphincter, with fluoroscopy enables the clinician to gather information about the pressure changes in the upper esophageal sphincter, as well as about the adequacy of pressure generation within the pharynx (from manometry), in addition to data on bolus and structural movements (from fluoroscopy). Combining manometry with fluoroscopy allows the clinician to be sure of the location of the manometric sensors in relation to the location of the bolus throughout the swallow.

Solid-state manometric sensors are used most often. These are positioned within a flexible catheter approximately 2.5 mm in diameter. The catheter usually contains two to three strain-gauge pressure sensors, so that when the tube is positioned in the pharynx, as shown in Figure 6.4, the most inferior sensor is in the esophagus, the middle sensor is in the cricopharyngeal region or just above, and the highest sensor is at the base of the tongue. The catheter containing the three pressure sensors is placed via radiography so that the exact location of the sensors can be noted. With the manometric sensors in place, a traditional videofluorographic study can be completed, using various bolus volumes and consistencies. The radiographic study is recorded on videotape, while the manometric data are recorded on a polygraph or high-fidelity data tape for later analysis. Timing information is recorded on the videotape and concurrently on one channel of the polygraph or data tape recorder, facilitating temporal synchronization of all data. This type of evaluation is highly people- and equipment-intensive and is not used in most evaluations of dysphagic patients. Rather, it is used selectively for patients who exhibit significant residual food remaining in the lower pharynx after the swallow, which may be indicative of problems in opening the

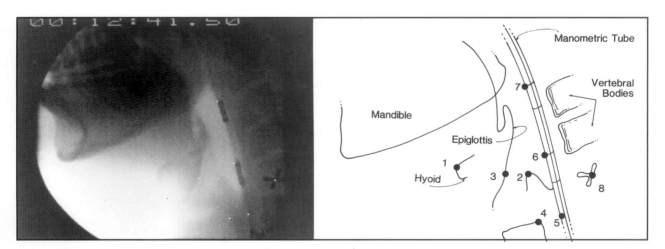

FIGURE 6.4. A lateral videoprint of the oral cavity and pharynx with a manometric tube in place, containing three rectangular metal manometric or pressure sensors. The top sensor is located opposite the tongue base, while the middle sensor is located just above the pyriform sinus. The inferior sensor is located just in the cervical esophagus. White dots identify structures of interest. Each structure is labeled on the right.

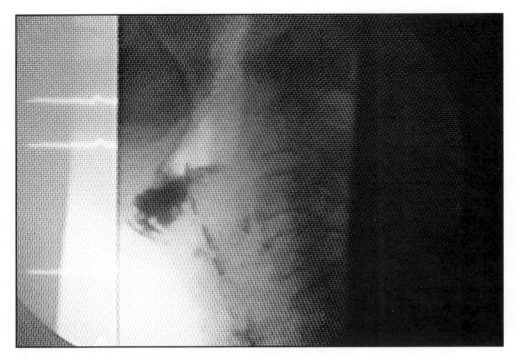

FIGURE 6.5. A lateral radiographic view of the oral cavity and pharynx of a patient undergoing manofluorography, with the pressure tracing superimposed on the radiographic image on the left.

cricopharyngeal region or in generating adequate pharyngeal pressure. Using combined manometry and videofluoroscopy, it is possible to identify problems with the cricopharyngeal muscle (from manometry), abnormalities in movement of the larynx to open the sphincter (from videofluoroscopy), and difficulty in generating adequate bolus pressure (from manometry).

Manofluorography

Another technique that combines manometry and fluoroscopy is manofluorography, a procedure developed by Dr. Fred McConnel at Emory University (Cerenko, McConnel, & Jackson, 1989). In this procedure, data are collected in the same way as described previously, with manometric sensors positioned radiographically and the videofluorographic study completed simultaneously with manometric data collection. However, data recording is completed using a split-screen video technique that allows the manometric tracings to be superimposed on the radiographic image, as shown in Figure 6.5. In this way, the examiner can see the pressures being generated at each sensor and the movements of the oropharyngeal structures generating these pressures, as well as the location of the bolus. Data recording and analysis is computerized. Manofluorography usually examines only 10-ml boluses, since that bolus volume is required to surround the pressure sensors consistently and allows the most accurate measurement of intrabolus pressures. Intrabolus pressure is the pressure within the bolus itself as the bolus is being driven through the pharynx. In manofluorography, specific forces generated during the pharyngeal swallow are calculated using the computer analysis.

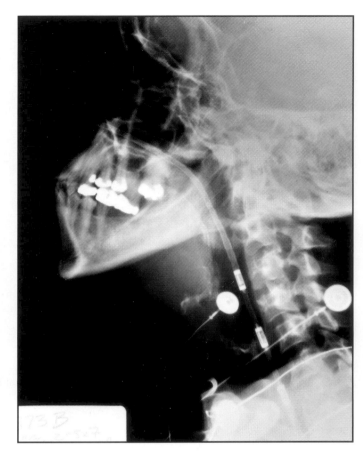

FIGURE 6.6. A lateral radiographic view of a patient with a manometric tube in place, containing three metal sensors and two surface electrodes on the neck.

Electromyography and Videofluorography

Electromyography (EMG) has also been combined with fluoroscopy to define the timing and duration of the firing of various muscle groups in relation to structural and bolus movements during the oropharyngeal swallow. The muscle groups most frequently studied are the submandibular and supralaryngeal (laryngeal elevator) muscles. In surface EMG, surface electrodes are placed over the muscles in question and glued in place by electrode collars. Each electrode is attached to an amplifier and, from the amplifier, to one channel of a recording device (polygraph or FM recorder). Timing information is also recorded concurrently on the polygraph or FM recorder and on the videofluoroscopic recording to allow temporal synchronization. Simultaneous videofluoroscopy and EMG are usually done for research purposes. However, surface EMG alone could be used as a biofeedback tool to monitor laryngeal elevation during swallow.

EMG, manometry, and fluoroscopy can all be combined, as shown in Figure 6.6. Combining these techniques allows measurement of pressures during swallowing (manometry), movement of food and structures during swallowing (fluoroscopy), and onset and termination of muscle activity (surface EMG). Currently, all of these combined technologies are used more often for research than for clinical care. However, in years to come, these combined procedures may be found useful, if not essential, in defining some types of dysphagia.

CHAPTER 7

Decision Making During
the Radiographic Study

This chapter presents a series of *decision trees* that represent the clinician's ongoing clinical decision-making process within the videofluorographic study of oropharyngeal swallow. A major goal of the radiographic procedure with dysphagic patients is to identify management strategies that will reduce the effects of the dysphagia, that is, eliminate aspiration and/or improve the efficiency of the swallow (Rasley et al., in press). Thus, when a patient exhibits either aspiration or severely inefficient swallowing during the X-ray study, the clinician should determine the anatomic or physiologic etiology of these symptoms and introduce selected treatment strategies within the X-ray session to improve or eliminate them. The treatment strategy used with a particular patient is selected to match the patient's swallowing physiology. As discussed earlier in this book, these interventions involve postural changes, increased sensory input, swallowing maneuvers, and food consistency (dietary) changes (Logemann, 1983; Rasley et al., in press). This chapter is designed to provide the clinician with examples of the ways in which these kinds of strategies are integrated into the radiographic study for various types of patients.

For each decision tree, there is an accompanying narrative that describes the thought process it represents. These examples are not meant to be prescriptions, but rather to represent examples of the clinician's thought process in evaluating the patient and planning treatment. Introducing treatment strategies in X Ray provides the clinician with data regarding the efficacy of the treatment procedures for the patient's particular swallowing problems. In a sense, it represents an individual treatment trial in which the strategies introduced can be evaluated objectively. It also provides an excellent teaching tool for the clinician to use with the patient, family, medical staff, and other caregivers to help them understand the importance of using these strategies as the patient eats, and the need for them to monitor such things as the patient's posture during mealtimes.

These examples are also not meant to be exhaustive. There are many other combinations of interventions that the clinician may wish to try with individual patients, and other types of swallowing disorders that can benefit from interventions in addition to those selected for illustration here. The kinds of treatment strategies introduced during the radiographic study and the order of their introduction will depend upon the patient's swallowing disorder and medical status, including his or her behavior, alertness, fatigue, and overall ability to follow directions and respond. As described earlier, usually selected postural techniques are attempted first, followed by increased sensory input, then swallowing maneuvers, and finally dietary changes, as appropriate.

Introduction of therapy strategies into the radiographic study may increase the number of swallows on which the patient aspirates, if none of the interventions is successful. If the volume of material given to the patient is small and measured, and the patient is able to cough reflexively or upon request and clear aspirated material after each aspiration event, the risk of pulmonary problems is minimal. The potential benefit to the patient in maintaining more oral intake and more normal dietary choices if the treatment strategies are successful usually far outweighs this minimal risk. However, there may be patients for whom any additional risk, however minimal, is unacceptable, such as the ventilator-dependent spinal-cord-injured patient or the patient with pulmonary disease or recent aspiration pneumonia. For these patients, the clinician may want to introduce only one selected intervention strategy, using a small (1- to 3-ml) bolus volume.

Apraxia of Swallow or Delayed Oral Onset of Swallow

The decision tree shown in Figure 7.1 represents the types of increased sensation that might be introduced in a patient with a swallowing apraxia who displays delayed oral onset of the swallow or delayed OTTs with searching lingual motions. A patient with a left cortical stroke may exhibit such problems. On the first swallow of 1 ml of liquid, the patient exhibits a highly inefficient 20-sec OTT. When downward pressure with the spoon is increased during presentation of the second 1-ml liquid bolus, the transit time is reduced to 10 sec. Introduction of a cold bolus reduces the transit time to 6 sec. The combination of increased pressure on the tongue and the cold bolus results in the most normal oral transit time (3 sec). This combination of cold and pressure is continued with larger bolus volumes. Self-feeding may also have been attempted to improve the swallow.

When switching food consistencies, the clinician may wish to observe another swallow with no additional sensory input, to determine whether the increased viscosity provides enough additional sensation so that cold and pressure are not needed. If oral transit slows again, cold and pressure can be reintroduced. For some patients, chewing provides additional sensory input and "breaks up" apraxic behavior.

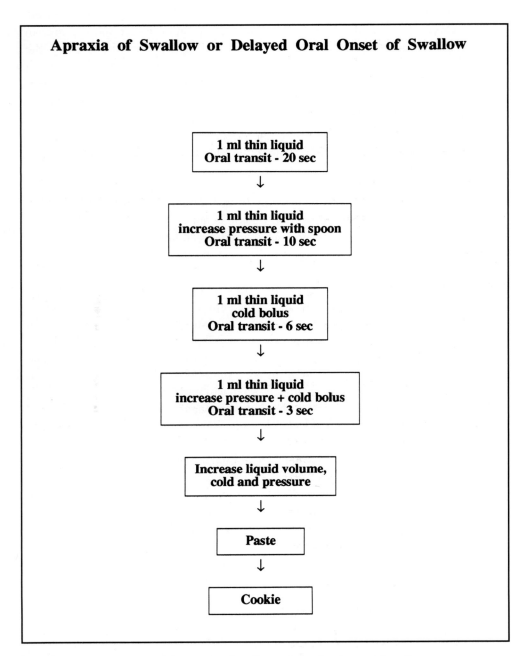

FIGURE 7.1. Decision tree for apraxia of swallow or delayed oral onset of swallow.

Reduced Range of Tongue Motion

The decision tree in Figure 7.2 represents a patient who has had a 50% glossectomy for oral cancer and who at one month postoperatively exhibits a reduced range of vertical motion of the tongue during the oral phase of swallow. When 1 ml of liquid is placed in the mouth, the patient loses control of the liquid and it spills prematurely into the pharynx and into the open airway, causing aspiration before the swallow. To eliminate this aspiration, the patient's head is tilted slightly forward to place the epiglottic angle more protectively over the airway. With the patient's head in the modified chin-down position, two 1-ml liquid swallows are repeated to demonstrate that this posture eliminates aspiration. If the patient is not able to propel the small (1-ml) volume backward with the chin slightly down, a 3-ml volume may be given or the 1 ml may be placed more posteriorly in the mouth. The patient's head cannot be tilted fully downward because of the tongue impairment; the full chin-down posture would make it difficult for the patient to clear the food from the mouth.

Following two 1-ml liquid swallows, the patient is given two swallows each of 3-, 5-, and 10-ml liquid boluses, thickened liquids in 3-ml amounts, and two boluses of 1/2 teaspoon of pudding or paste material. Cookie is not given, as this patient cannot yet chew because of the reduced tongue mass and reduced lateral tongue motion postoperatively. If the head tilted forward eliminates aspiration on all of these volumes of liquid, thick liquid, and paste, the study will then be terminated. However, if the head tilted forward does not eliminate aspiration, the clinician will stop the X-ray study and teach the patient (while in X Ray) to use the supraglottic swallow in order to protect the airway before and during the swallow. After several trials, when the patient has learned the supraglottic swallow, the clinician will present small to large volumes of thin liquid, thick liquid, and paste materials. If the patient aspirates on any volume despite the head being tilted forward or introduction of the supraglottic swallow, or a combination of these two techniques, the clinician will move from thin liquids to thick liquids and paste materials. Patients with a reduced tongue range of motion or control often have the greatest difficulty with thin liquids, which splash and move by gravity alone. They usually have less difficulty controlling thicker liquids. Paste materials may be difficult for these patients because greater tongue pressure is needed to propel thick foods through the oral cavity.

At the end of the radiographic study of this patient, the clinician (swallowing therapist) should indicate the conditions under which the patient can successfully take oral nutrition, including the best types and volumes of food, as well as the therapy techniques that are necessary.

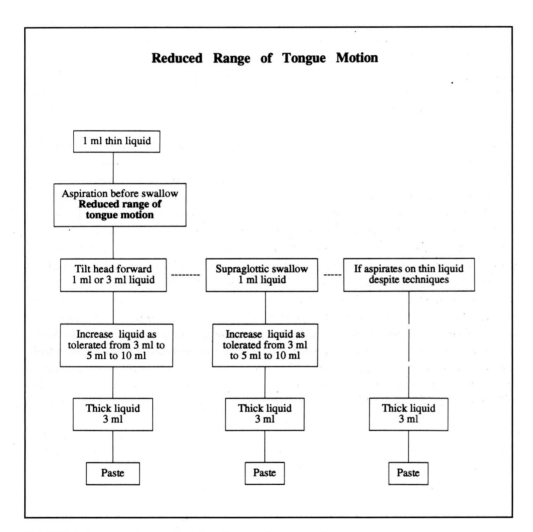

FIGURE 7.2. Decision tree for reduced range of tongue motion.

Delayed Triggering of the Pharyngeal Swallow

Patients with delay in triggering the pharyngeal swallow often complain of difficulty taking thin liquids orally. It is not uncommon for the patient to aspirate before the swallow on even a small volume of thin liquid, such as 1 ml, because the liquid splashes into the pharynx while the airway is still open before the pharyngeal swallow is triggered, and the liquid quickly falls into the open airway. As shown in Figure 7.3, to reduce the chance of liquid entering the airway during the delay, the patient's chin would be tilted downward to narrow the airway entrance, put the epiglottis in a more protective position, and widen the valleculae (Welch et al., 1993). With the patient's head in the chin-down position, two swallows of 1 ml of liquid should be attempted again. If the two 1-ml swallows are successful, the clinician should proceed to two swallows each of 3, 5, and 10 ml and cup drinking of thin liquid, as tolerated, that is, if aspiration is eliminated. Then, pureed food and cookie should be given. The patient may not need to use the chin-down posture during swallows of thicker foods. Whether or not the clinician asks the patient to use the chin-down posture on all swallows will depend on the severity of the patient's pharyngeal delay (longer delay, greater use of a chin-down posture), and on the patient's compliance and ease of learning to use the chin-down posture. If the patient is easily confused by changing directions, it is usually best to maintain the chin-down posture on all swallows of all food consistencies.

If the patient aspirates again at any volume of thin liquids despite the chin-down posture, the clinician may wish to teach the patient to protect the airway voluntarily by holding the breath (the supraglottic swallow). Then the same thin liquid volume on which the patient aspirated should be presented again. If the supraglottic swallow protects the airway adequately on smaller volumes of liquid, the clinician should progress through larger volumes to assure that the patient can take more normal amounts of liquid and still protect the airway. From there, the clinician can proceed to thicker foods and cookie materials. If the supraglottic swallow is not successful in eliminating aspiration alone or in combination with the chin-down posture, the clinician may wish to move from thin liquids to thickened liquids of small to large volumes and then to purees and cookie. Patients with a delayed pharyngeal swallow are usually able to swallow food of a thicker consistency more easily.

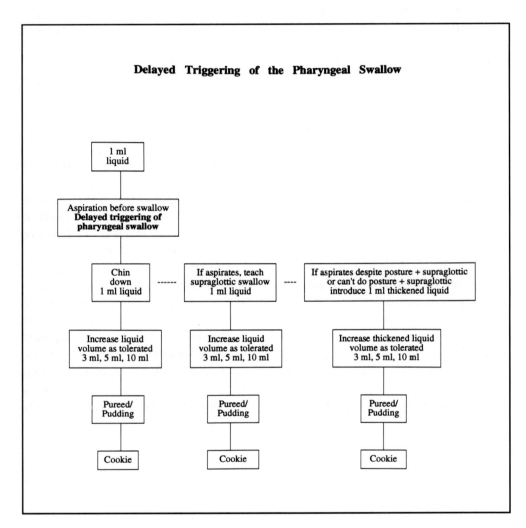

FIGURE 7.3.   Decision tree for delayed triggering of the pharyngeal swallow.

Reduced Closure of the Laryngeal Vestibule (Airway Entrance)

Some patients exhibit failure to close the larynx at the vestibule, that is, the airway entrance between the arytenoid and the posterior wall of the base of the epiglottis. The decision tree for this type of patient is shown in Figure 7.4. Material then enters the laryngeal vestibule during the swallow (laryngeal penetration) and is prevented from going lower in the airway by closure at the level of the true vocal folds, as illustrated in Figure 7.5. Unless this material is cleared from the laryngeal vestibule as the larynx continues to elevate and close during the swallow, this penetrated material is often aspirated after the swallow when the patient opens the airway to breathe. If the patient aspirates after the swallow because of reduced closure of the laryngeal vestibule, the patient may be placed in a chin-down posture to improve airway protection by increasing epiglottic overhang and narrowing the airway entrance (Welch et al., 1993). Small volumes of liquid should be given, and if aspiration is eliminated with the postural change, the volume of liquid should be increased from 3 ml to 5 ml to 10 ml, then to cup drinking, as tolerated. Then paste and cookie should be given.

If the chin-down posture does not eliminate aspiration, the clinician may wish to teach the patient the supersupraglottic swallow. This technique is designed to voluntarily close the entrance to the airway at the arytenoid–epiglottic base level. The patient can be taught this technique quickly in X Ray and reevaluated to define its effectiveness. After learning the technique, the patient should be given small to large volumes of liquid, followed by paste and masticated material, as tolerated.

The Mendelsohn maneuver may also be used with this patient because reduced closure of the laryngeal vestibule may result from reduced laryngeal elevation. In some people, laryngeal elevation brings the arytenoid cartilage physically closer to the epiglottic base, so that less arytenoid tilting is required to contact the epiglottic base and achieve closure of the vestibule. The Mendelsohn maneuver can be taught while the patient is in X Ray. Again, small to large volumes of liquid can be presented, as tolerated, followed by thickened liquid, paste, and cookie materials as tolerated, that is, as long as aspiration is eliminated.

If none of these strategies successfully improves swallowing on liquids, advancing to thicker foods may eliminate the aspiration. Thicker foods sometimes slide past the airway entrance without entering the vestibule.

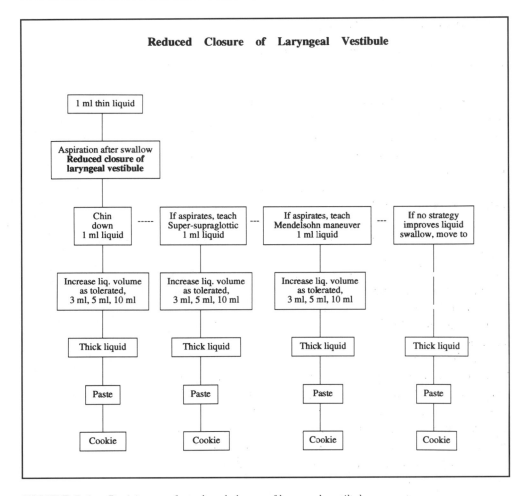

FIGURE 7.4.   Decision tree for reduced closure of laryngeal vestibule.

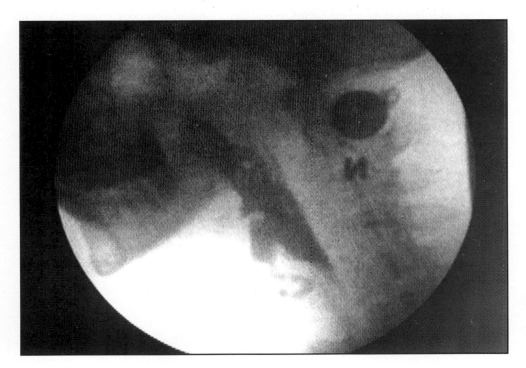

FIGURE 7.5.   A lateral videoprint of the oral cavity and pharynx in a patient with reduced closure of the airway entrance but good vocal fold closure. Barium has entered the airway entrance to the surface of the vocal folds.

Reduced Laryngeal Closure

The decision tree in Figure 7.6 shows a patient with reduced laryngeal closure. These patients fail to accomplish closure at any level of laryngeal valving from the entrance of the airway through and including the true vocal folds. Thus, they aspirate during the pharyngeal swallow, as material enters the airway and proceeds below the vocal folds. When this occurs, the clinician can put the patient's head in the chin-down posture to increase epiglottic protection of the airway and diminish the width of the airway opening. Presentation of small to large volumes of liquid as tolerated will identify the largest volume for which this technique continues to maintain airway protection.

If this technique does not prevent entrance of material into the trachea, the clinician may try head rotation, which applies extrinsic pressure to the thyroid cartilage, thus pushing one vocal fold toward midline to improve closure of the airway. Head rotation to each side may be examined, though usually the side of known laryngeal weakness (paresis) should be attempted first. Again, liquid swallows from small to large volumes should be given as tolerated to identify the volumes at which this technique succeeds in eliminating all aspiration. If head rotation alone does not improve the swallow, combining head rotation with the chin-down posture may provide sufficient protection. Again, various volumes and food consistencies should be tested as tolerated.

If the combined postural techniques do not facilitate airway protection and prevent aspiration during the swallow, the supraglottic swallow may be attempted. For this technique, the patient is taught to voluntarily close the airway before and during the swallow. The supraglottic swallow usually increases the strength of closure of the larynx. If neither the postural techniques nor the supraglottic swallow is successful in eliminating aspiration on thin liquids, the clinician may advance to foods of thicker consistency. Foods of greater viscosity may slide past the airway entrance rather than entering the airway.

At the end of this radiographic session, the clinician should have identified the techniques that best eliminate aspiration and make it possible for the patient to eat at least some selected food consistencies and volumes.

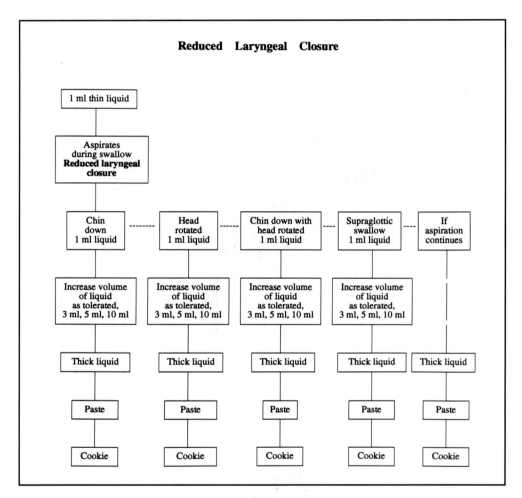

FIGURE 7.6.   Decision tree for reduced laryngeal closure.

Unilateral Pharyngeal Weakness

Patients with unilateral pharyngeal weakness exhibit asymmetrical residue (greater on one side of the pharynx than the other). The decision tree for such a patient is shown in Figure 7.7. These patients usually have greater difficulty swallowing larger volumes of liquid and thicker foods. They may be able to manage 1- and 3-ml volumes of liquid with only mild to moderate amounts of residue in the pharynx after the swallow, but on 5- or 10-ml volumes, there may be significant residue. These patients need to be examined in the P-A view to determine whether or not the residue is on only one side of the pharynx. As the volume increases and the residue increases in the pharynx, the patient may aspirate after the swallow, as material on the one side of the pharynx is inhaled into the airway. With a unilateral pharyngeal weakness, head rotation toward the weaker side should be attempted, thus eliminating the weaker side of the pharynx from the bolus path. Then larger volumes of liquid may be introduced while continuing to keep the head rotated. If the patient continues to swallow without aspiration, the clinician may wish to present paste and masticated materials. If at some point in the series of liquid swallows the patient aspirates again, the patient may be taught to cough and clear the residue before opening the airway after the swallow.

When the patient has learned this sequence, the study may be continued with larger volumes of liquid, paste, and masticated materials, as desired. If the patient has difficulty learning to cough and clear the residue before it is aspirated, double swallows may be attempted. In this technique, the patient swallows twice in a row on each bolus, thus clearing more of the residue. If head rotation and the other techniques are not solving the problem, the clinician may wish to introduce the side-lying posture, with the patient lying on the side corresponding to the stronger side of the pharynx. The head should be slightly supported so that the cervical vertebrae are in line with the thoracic vertebrae. In this position, the patient may again be given swallows of increasingly larger volumes of liquid, paste, and cookie materials. Lying down changes the direction of the gravitational effect on the bolus, tending to keep residue in the pharynx rather than dropping it down the airway and thus decreasing the chance of aspiration after the swallow.

If no aspiration occurs, but the residue increases with successive food swallows, alternating liquid and food swallows may be attempted to "wash" residual food through the pharynx. Or alternating food swallows and dry swallows may be successful in clearing the residue.

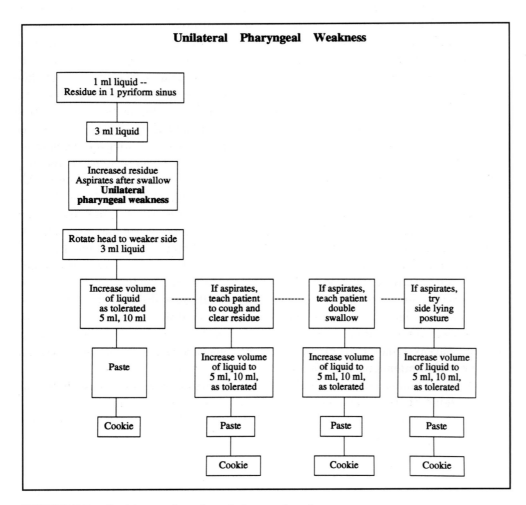

FIGURE 7.7.   Decision tree for unilateral pharyngeal weakness.

Reduced Hyoid and Anterior Laryngeal Movement and Cricopharyngeal Dysfunction

Some patients exhibit reduced hyoid and laryngeal movement forward and upward during the swallow, which reduces the extent and/or duration of cricopharyngeal opening, since laryngeal anterior movement controls a large portion of cricopharyngeal opening (Jacob et al., 1989). Patients with this disorder often exhibit greater problems swallowing thickened foods than liquids. However, they may exhibit a severely inefficient swallow, even on small volumes of liquid, which results in significant residue in the pyriform sinuses after the swallow. Many patients with reduced laryngeal motion also exhibit a unilateral pharyngeal weakness. When this combination of problems is noted, the decision three shown in Figure 7.8 may be used. The clinician may want to first introduce head rotation to the weaker side of the pharynx, which eliminates the weaker side of the pharynx from the bolus path, increases bolus pressure, and thereby increases the width of cricopharyngeal opening (Jacob et al., 1989). If head rotation does not facilitate cricopharyngeal opening, the Mendelsohn maneuver may be taught to the patient. The Mendelsohn maneuver is designed to prolong and extend laryngeal elevation voluntarily and, thereby, to prolong cricopharyngeal opening. If this technique does not result in prolonged cricopharyngeal opening and more efficient swallowing, the clinician may want to combine head rotation with the Mendelsohn maneuver.

Whichever technique or techniques work best, the clinician will want to increase the volume of liquids swallowed (two to three swallows of each volume) as tolerated, and then move to paste and masticated materials as tolerated. If the patient aspirates on any swallow and continues to aspirate despite these techniques, the study should be discontinued and therapy begun. Most patients with cricopharyngeal dysfunction secondary to reduced laryngeal movement, such as those with brain-stem strokes or spinal cord injuries who have undergone anterior spinal fusion, exhibit recovery of swallow over time. Usually, most recover within 1 to 6 months. In most cases, cricopharyngeal myotomy has been found to be unsuccessful in improving swallowing in these patients because their swallowing disorder is related to reduced laryngeal movement, not failure of the cricopharyngeal muscle to relax. It is important that time be allowed for recovery before any surgical intervention is contemplated.

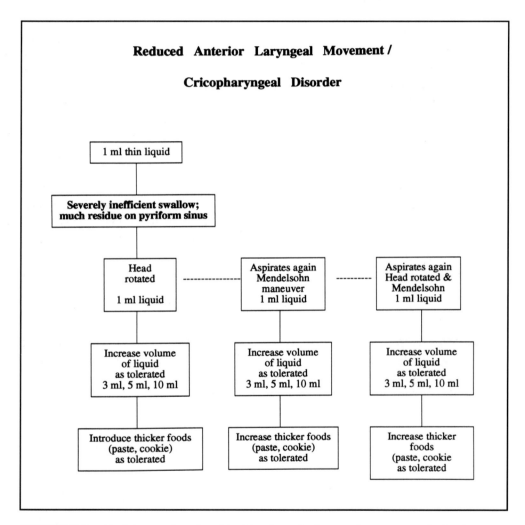

FIGURE 7.8.   Decision tree for reduced hyoid and anterior laryngeal movement and cricopharyngeal dysfunction.

NOTES

Report and Recommendations

When the MBS is completed, the clinician will summarize the results in a report that should include:

- Any relevant background information and history
- A description of the patient's oropharyngeal anatomy and swallowing physiology
- The effects of treatment strategies attempted
- Recommendations for method of nutritional intake
- The need for and nature of therapy
- The need and schedule for reevaluation
- The need for other assessments or consultations

Relevant Background and History

If the patient is an outpatient, relevant medical history, including the presence and status of any airway maintenance devices such as a tracheostomy and any nonoral feeding procedures, should be included in the report. If the patient is an inpatient, relevant aspects of the patient's medical status, such as the presence of a tracheostomy, mechanical ventilation, and the nature of any nonoral feeding present, should be included.

Description of the Swallow Function

The report should contain a description of the oral stage of the swallow, including:

- The speed of the oral stage of swallow (OTTs)
- Any motility disorders causing slowed oral transit of the bolus or oral residue
- The cause, location, and approximate amount (percentage of the bolus) of any residue in the mouth
- The cause and approximate amount of any aspiration seen before or during the oral stage of the swallow

Normalcy of triggering of the pharyngeal swallow should be described, including:

- An estimate (measure) of the duration of any delay in triggering the pharyngeal swallow
- The location of the bolus in the pharynx during the delay
- The occurrence of any aspiration during the delay

Finally, the pharyngeal stage of swallow should be described, including:

- PTT
- The location and approximate amount (percentage of the bolus) of any residual food in the pharynx after the swallow
- The movement disorder causing the residue, such as, reduced tongue-base retraction or reduced laryngeal elevation
- The presence and approximate amount (percentage of the bolus) of any aspiration during the pharyngeal stage of the swallow because of reduced airway closure
- The presence, approximate amount (percentage of the bolus), and etiology of any aspiration after the swallow occurring when residue remains in the pharynx after the swallow and enters the airway during inhalation after the swallow

If swallows of all consistencies exhibit the same disorders, this can be indicated at the beginning of the report. If the disorders vary by food consistency, the report sequence should be repeated for each food consistency.

Recommendations

The report should also indicate the effects of any trial therapy or compensatory strategies evaluated and make recommendations regarding (a) potential therapy for the patient, (b) suggestions for nutritional management, and (c) the recommended schedule for any reevaluation.

Effects of Treatment Strategies

The effects of any trial therapy techniques attempted during the radiographic study should be described. If no effect is seen, a simple sentence can be used such as "Postural techniques and the supraglottic swallow were unsuccessful in eliminating aspiration." If therapy techniques are successful, the conditions under which the patient can eat successfully should be defined, for example: "With the chin down and head rotated to the left, aspiration is eliminated on all volumes and food consistencies. Recommend eating orally only with the chin down and head rotated," "Using the Mendelsohn maneuver, laryngeal movement and cricopharyngeal opening are improved enough so that 3 ml (spoonful) of thin liquid can be given orally in therapy only."

Suggestions for Nutritional Management

Recommendations regarding method of nutritional intake are usually made using two guidelines: (a) speed of the swallow and (b) amount of aspiration seen across the various consistencies of food swallowed and under the various treatment conditions introduced.

Speed of the Swallow. Speed of the swallow is defined as combined oral and pharyngeal transit times. If these combined transit times are more than 10 sec (five times longer than normal oral plus pharyngeal transit time of 2 sec) for all consistencies of food swallowed, it is unlikely that the patient will be able to maintain sufficient nutrition and hydration by mouth to sustain health. Often, dysphagic patients will fatigue before they achieve adequate oral intake. If even one food consistency can be swallowed in 10 sec or less, the patient can usually be given sufficient caloric supplements in this single consistency to maintain adequate oral nutrition and hydration. The patient who cannot swallow any food consistency in less than 10 sec can eat as much as possible orally, but will need nutritional supplements presented by some nonoral method.

In addition to measuring the speed of the swallow in the radiographic study, the clinician should assess the overall feeding situation in patients who have dysphagia resulting from cerebral palsy or other neuromotor disorders. These patients not only may eat slowly, but may lose so much food from the mouth that only a very small amount of food passes to the back of the oral cavity to be swallowed. Patients such as these, whose speed of swallow is borderline (e.g., 9 sec) and who are losing significant amounts of food from the mouth, will probably not get sufficient nutrition or hydration by mouth and will need nonoral supplementation. It is important to emphasize again that these patients can take as much oral nutrition as they are able or wish to because they are not aspirating. The critical issue in these patients is maintaining adequate nutrition and hydration.

Amount of aspiration. The second criterion in recommending oral versus nonoral feeding is the *amount of aspiration.* As a general guideline, if a patient aspirates more than 10% of all food consistencies despite the introduction of treatment strategies, he or she should not be eating by mouth, but should instead be receiving therapy directed toward alleviating or eliminating the cause of aspiration, and should receive nonoral nutrition and hydration. There is no evidence that patients will benefit from being fed when they aspirate excessively, even with a tracheostomy tube in place with the cuff inflated. This latter procedure does not directly treat the aspiration, and it puts the patient at risk for tracheal irritation and possible development of a TE fistula from vertical rubbing of the inflated tracheostomy cuff against the tracheal wall. Those patients who aspirate on all foods despite the therapy strategies introduced in the radiographic study should be recommended for complete nonoral intake. Those who aspirate during the radiographic study on only one food consistency can eat other consistencies orally, eliminating the consistency (e.g., thin liquid) on which they aspirate. Or, if the patient aspirates during the radiographic study, but postural changes or other treatment strategies eliminate the aspiration as documented radiographically, the patient can eat those foods on which aspiration was eliminated using the intervention strategies.

The 10% criterion is only applicable to patients who reliably cough when they aspirate, consistently clear the aspirated material, and have not had any pulmonary complications such as pneumonia. In general, clinicians should not recommend oral intake for patients who are aspirating consistently any amount if they are older (over age 80), immobile, or have pulmonary problems, unless the aspiration can be stopped with strategies as demonstrated radiographically.

Some patients who aspirate less than 10% should not be eating. If a patient is aspirating even small amounts of food but does not cough or respond to the aspiration, cannot cough well, or has pulmonary complications, and the aspiration is not stopped by treatment strategies, nonoral feeding should usually be recommended.

Recommended Therapy Procedures

These procedures will depend on the nature of the swallowing motility disorders and the underlying cause of the patient's swallowing disorder, for example, stroke, head trauma, or progressive neurologic disease. Recommendations for therapy strategies should focus on the purpose of the therapy, for example, therapy to improve laryngeal elevation, closure at the airway entrance, or triggering of the pharyngeal swallow.

Recommended Schedule for Reevaluation

The recommended schedule for reevaluation will depend on the patient's medical diagnosis, anticipated rate of recovery, and prognosis. For the neurologic patient in the process of recovery, reevaluation in 3–4 weeks is often appropriate. For the patient with a degenerative neurologic condition, reevaluation in 3–6 months, or sooner should worsening of swallowing symptoms occur, is frequently adequate. At times, a statement such as "Reevaluation is suggested when clinical improvement is seen" is most accurate. In this way, the clinician working with the patient can determine when the patient has made sufficient progress to warrant a reevaluation. In general, reevaluation should be done when the patient is ready for a major advance in treatment, such as moving from nonoral to oral intake.

Recommendations for Other Consultations or Assessments

These recommendations are sometimes needed, based on the results of the MBS. This is usually true if the patient has dysphagia with no known medical diagnosis or if the patient has suspected esophageal disorders. The patient with oropharyngeal swallowing disorders and no known medical diagnosis or etiology must be referred to the full dysphagia team for assessment and diagnosis. In our experience, these patients most often have a neurologic disease such as motor neuron disease, Parkinson's disease, myasthenia gravis, or brain tumors. The diagnosis is critical for appropriate overall management of the patient and the patient's swallowing disorder. In some of these patients—for example, those with Parkinson's disease or myasthenia gravis—medication for their neurologic disease can significantly improve or eliminate their swallowing disorder, thus eliminating the need for swallowing therapy. In other cases, such as motor neuron disease, the diagnosis will dictate the nature of treatment. Motor neuron patients do not benefit from direct exercise programs because of fatigue; they should be treated instead with compensatory strategies that do not create fatigue.

The patient with suspected esophageal disorders should be referred to a gastroenterologist for further assessment and management. Esophageal disorders may be suspected because of patient complaints (burning in the throat or chest, pressure or discomfort in the chest, gagging or coughing toward the end or after a meal, waking up at night gagging or coughing, or a chronic bad taste in the mouth) or because backflow of liquid or food from the esophagus into the pharynx is observed during the radiographic study.

In summary, the report of the radiographic study should clearly describe the patient's swallowing problems, effects of treatment strategies, and recommendations for further assessment and management of the disorders and oral and nonoral intake.

CHAPTER 9

Sample Reports

NOTES

Anumber of sample reports from modified barium swallows are presented in this chapter, with the intent of indicating the types of information generally included. As can be seen, aspiration is always defined according to when it occurs in relationship to the pharyngeal stage of swallowing (i.e., before, during, or after). Also, an estimate of the amount of aspiration occurring on swallows of particular food consistencies is noted. Effects of treatment strategies are defined. Recommendations for therapy follow the description of the swallowing disorders in each case, as do recommendations for oral versus nonoral feeding. It is important to remember that the ultimate decisions regarding feeding-and-management strategies are determined by the patient's attending physician. It is the swallowing therapist's responsibility to provide the attending physician with a maximum amount of accurate information regarding the patient's swallowing physiology so that the attending physician can make an educated decision regarding the patient's management.

You will note that most reports focus on the major disorders and their management. In writing reports, brevity and clarity are desired to ensure that the most important points are conveyed to the reader.

Inpatient Evaluation Reports

Inpatient evaluations are usually written directly in the patient's medical chart at the time of the radiographic study and are shorter than outpatient evaluations, which include identifying and descriptive history data. Several inpatient reports are provided to illustrate descriptions of various disorders and recommendations.

Inpatient Evaluation: Normal

Modified barium swallow completed. Results show normal oral and pharyngeal transit times with no motility disorders. No aspiration was seen and no residue remained in the oral cavity or pharynx after any swallow of liquid, paste, or masticated material. Summary: Essentially normal swallow.

Inpatient Evaluation: Oral-Phase Disorders, Pharyngeal Phase Normal

Modified barium swallow completed. Results show severely reduced oromotor control and delayed initiation of the swallow orally. Lip closure was reduced bilaterally. Vertical lingual movement was reduced. No lingual lateralization or vertical mashing on chewing attempts was seen so the patient cannot handle foods requiring mastication. The pharyngeal swallow is triggered well but external signs of triggering

147

are poor because of reduced hyoid-bone movement. Once the pharyngeal swallow is triggered, the pharynx empties well (no residue) and no aspiration is seen. This patient's swallowing problem is limited to the oral phase of the swallow. Suggest limiting diet to liquid and pureed foods requiring no chewing. Will initiate therapy to improve lingual elevation and lateralization.

Inpatient Evaluation: Focus on the Pharyngeal Phase

Modified barium swallow completed. Oral transit times are normal for all bolus types with no motility problems. The pharyngeal swallow was triggered well. When the pharyngeal swallow was triggered, there was residual food (50% of each bolus) in the valleculae and on the pharyngeal walls, indicating reduced tongue-base posterior movement and reduced pharyngeal-wall contraction. Residue remained the same on all swallows of all foods. No aspiration occurred. Alternating liquid and food swallows to clear the residue was successful. Suggest this strategy with full oral intake. Recommend therapy to improve tongue-base posterior movement. No reevaluation is needed.

Inpatient Evaluation Followed by Outpatient Reassessment: Head-Injured Four-Year-Old Child with Unilateral Pharyngeal Damage and Reduced Laryngeal Movement

First inpatient evaluation. Modified barium swallow completed. Results show normal oral transit times with no motility problems. The pharyngeal swallow was triggered 2 to 3 sec late. During the delay, the bolus routinely remained in the valleculae. When the pharyngeal swallow was triggered, reduced anterior and vertical laryngeal movement was seen, causing reduced opening of the cricopharyngeal region. Residue remained in one of the pyriform sinuses and on one pharyngeal wall, indicating a unilateral pharyngeal-wall dysfunction. Only approximately 20% of a liquid bolus entered the esophagus. No thicker food entered the esophagus. The remainder of the bolus was left in the pyriform sinuses and fell into the airway after the swallow. No cough was elicited in response to this aspiration. The patient was asked to turn the head to the damaged side of the pharynx to eliminate the damaged side of the pharynx from the bolus path. This strategy resulted in improved clearance of 1-ml and 3-ml liquid boluses (approximately 50–75% of each bolus entered the esophagus with no aspiration after the swallow). On 5-ml liquid boluses, increased residue and aspiration occurred. The Mendelsohn maneuver could not be attempted because of the child's age. Suggest continued nonoral feeding with reevaluation in 3 to 4 weeks to assess the progress of recovery. Also suggest thermal-tactile stimulation to improve the triggering of the pharyngeal swallow. One-ml and 3-ml amounts of liquid can be introduced in therapy.

Second inpatient evaluation. Modified barium swallow completed. Results show normal oral transit times with no motility problems. The pharyngeal swallow was triggered normally. Laryngeal movement and cricopharyngeal opening have also improved, so that approximately 80% of each 1-ml to 10-ml liquid bolus and 20% of each pudding bolus enter the esophagus per swallow with the head in a normal position. With the head turned to one side, the entire liquid bolus (1 ml to 10 ml) entered the esophagus with no residue and no aspiration. Fifty percent of the pudding bolus entered the esophagus. Suggest liquids given orally with the head turned and continued nonoral feeding to maintain nutrition. Suggest reevaluation in 1 to 2 months.

Outpatient follow-up. [Name], a 5-year-old girl, of [address], was seen for videofluoroscopic examination of swallowing on July 18, 1983. During swallows of 1 ml to 10 ml of liquids and cup drinking of liquids, paste, and masticated material (cookie) with the head in a neutral position, oral transit times were normal with no motility problems. The pharyngeal swallow was triggered well. After the swallow, a very small amount of residue remained only in the left pyriform sinus.

At this time, [name] exhibits only a few minor signs of her previously severe swallowing problem. Full oral feeding on all food consistencies can be resumed. She should still be careful of eating too much in one bolus or of eating too fast. This information was given to [name] and her parents, who indicated that they agreed with these recommendations.

Inpatient Evaluation: Posthemilaryngectomy

[Name], a 48-year-old woman, of [address], was seen for videofluoroscopic examination of swallowing on March 10, 1985, 7 days after her hemilaryngectomy. [Name] has not attempted oral intake prior to this time.

Oral transit times were normal with no motility problems. The pharyngeal swallow was triggered well. When the pharyngeal swallow was triggered, pharyngeal transit times were normal. With the head in an upright position almost all of the bolus was aspirated during the pharyngeal swallow because of inadequate laryngeal closure. With the head down so that the epiglottis overhung the airway, no aspiration was seen on any swallows of any volume or consistency.

[Name] can begin oral feeding with the head down to prevent aspiration. This is a temporary compensatory procedure until [name] can achieve adequate laryngeal closure to protect the airway. Will initiate adduction exercises to improve laryngeal closure.

Outpatient Evaluation Reports

Of necessity, outpatient reports include patient identification information and any relevant history. In other ways, the content is similar to that of the inpatient reports. Included here are reports of a variety of patients including a patient who was reevaluated on several occasions, and reports of a variety of surgically treated head-and-neck-cancer patients. Also included is a detailed report of the swallowing and speech radiographic assessment of a total laryngectomee. In this special surgical group, the reconstructed pharyngoesophagus must function for both speech and swallowing, so that it is often helpful to the clinician to assess both functions radiographically if a total-laryngectomy patient (a) is having difficulty acquiring esophageal voice, (b) is a candidate for a surgical prosthetic voice-restoration technique, or (c) is having difficulty swallowing.

Outpatient Evaluation: Bilateral Cortical Stroke

[Name], a 67-year-old man, of [address], was seen for videofluoroscopic examination of swallowing on June 6, 1991. He had suffered a stroke about 2 years ago and has had trouble swallowing since then, although he has not lost weight and is eating a full diet orally. [Name] said his "throat" had been dilated about a month ago. He also said he coughs a lot when eating.

During swallows of liquid and paste, oral transit times were normal with no motility problems. The pharyngeal swallow was triggered 2 to 4 sec late, with greater delay on thicker foods. When the pharyngeal swallow was triggered, pharyngeal-wall contraction was reduced bilaterally, resulting in residue in the valleculae, pyriform sinuses, and pharyngeal walls. Tongue-base posterior movement was reduced, contributing to the vallecular residue. After the swallow some of this residue fell over into the airway, but [name] was successful in regularly and spontaneously expectorating it. It takes [name] three to four repeated swallows per bolus to clear the residue from the pharynx. This does not appear to be a problem with laryngeal elevation or a cricopharyngeal dysfunction as much as it is related to generally reduced tongue-base and pharyngeal-wall function. At this time, [name] appears to be maintaining his weight. Effortful swallow resulted in clearing more food on the first swallow of a bolus and the need for only one dry swallow to clear residue.

Suggest thermal-tactile stimulation of the pharyngeal swallow and use of the effortful swallow and alternation of liquid and solid foods to wash the pharynx clear of residue, with reevaluation in 1 to 2 months. Also suggest exercises to improve tongue-base posterior movement.

Outpatient Follow-up Evaluation: Poststroke

[Name], a 74-year-old woman, of [address], was seen for videofluoroscopic examination of oropharyngeal swallowing on August 8, 1992. [Name] suffered a right cortical stroke 3 months ago. She has been attempting small amounts of soft food in her swallowing practice but maintains nutrition by gastrostomy. She has been doing thermal-tactile stimulation of her pharyngeal swallow at home.

During videofluoroscopic examination of oropharyngeal swallow, oral transit times were only slightly slowed (2 sec) with mild reduction in vertical tongue movement. The pharyngeal swallow was triggered 3 to 4 sec late on 1- to 10-ml volumes of liquid. During the delay, the bolus collected in the valleculae. [Name] aspirated during the delay on 10 ml of liquid. The chin-down posture was introduced and aspiration was eliminated on 10-ml boluses and cup drinking of thin liquids. The delay was only 2 sec on soft foods (paste) and solid foods (cookie) with no aspiration. This is a significant improvement from previous studies where the delay was 8 to 10 sec on all volumes and viscosities. When the pharyngeal swallow was triggered, the pharynx emptied well. All motor elements of the pharyngeal swallow were normal. It was suggested to [name] that she begin oral intake on soft foods and take liquids with the chin down. In all likelihood, if her improvement continues she will be able to eliminate the gastrostomy in another 2 to 3 weeks. She was also directed to continue her thermal-tactile stimulation of the pharyngeal swallow. She should be reevaluated radiographically in 1 month.

Outpatient Evaluation: Brain-Stem Stroke—Three Weeks Poststroke

[Name], a 43-year-old woman, of [address], was seen for a videofluoroscopic examination of swallowing on February 20, 1991. [Name] has a gastrostomy for oral nutrition and hydration. Currently there is no oral intake.

During swallows of 1 ml of liquid, oral transit times were normal with no motility problems. The pharyngeal swallow was triggered 2 to 3 sec late. When the pharyngeal swallow was triggered, the larynx moved poorly, resulting in reduced cricopharyngeal opening. A posterior-anterior view revealed residue in one side of the pharynx (pyriform sinus), indicating a unilateral pharyngeal-wall weakness. Only 10% of the bolus was swallowed. Head rotation to the weak side of the pharynx resulted in improved pharyngeal clearance with 50% of the 1-ml boluses but only 25% of the 3-ml boluses being swallowed. After the 3-ml swallows there was aspiration of the residue. [Name] was taught the Mendelsohn maneuver, which resulted in increased laryngeal motion and cricopharyngeal opening with improved clearance of the bolus on 3 ml of liquid. On 5-ml boluses, aspiration after the swallow returned. When the Mendelsohn maneuver and head rotation were combined, 5-ml and 10-ml boluses were swallowed without aspiration. However, increased residue and aspiration occurred on pudding materials. Suggest continued practice of the Mendelsohn maneuver and head rotation with oral intake of thin liquids in up to 10-ml amounts. Suggest maintaining the gastrostomy to assure adequate nutrition and hydration. Suggest reevaluation in 3 to 4 weeks to assess improvement and return to full oral intake.

Outpatient Evaluation: Supraglottic Laryngectomy with Two Follow-Up Examinations

First outpatient evaluation.   [Name], a 60-year-old man, of [address], was seen for videofluoroscopic examination of oropharyngeal swallowing on March 23, 1992. [Name] underwent an extended supraglottic laryngectomy two weeks ago. He currently takes nutrition via a nasogastric tube.

During all swallows, oral transit times were normal with no motility problems. The pharyngeal swallow was triggered well. During the pharyngeal stage of the swallow, approximately 50% of the bolus was aspirated directly into the airway with no closure of the arytenoid to the base of the tongue or the vocal folds. A posterior-anterior view revealed the two vocal cords to be at the same height. The remaining 50% of the bolus collected in the pharynx because of reduced laryngeal elevation until it was expectorated. The supersupraglottic swallow was attempted and resulted in reduction of aspiration to 30% of the bolus.

Suggest practice with the supersupraglottic swallow to improve closure of the entrance to the airway (arytenoid to the base of the epiglottis) and continued nonoral feeding because of excessive aspiration.

First outpatient follow-up.   [Name], a 60-year-old man, of [address], was seen for videofluoroscopic examination of oropharyngeal swallowing on April 25, 1992. [Name] underwent an extended supraglottic laryngectomy six weeks ago and has been practicing the supersupraglottic swallow.

[Name] was using the supersupraglottic swallow during all swallows. Oral transit times were normal with no motility problems. The pharyngeal swallow was triggered well. During the pharyngeal stage of the swallow approximately 20% of the bolus was aspirated directly through the airway entrance and glottis, indicating improved but still incomplete closure of the airway entrance and vocal folds during the swallow. Of the remaining bolus, approximately half entered the esophagus and half remained in the pharynx after the swallow because of reduced laryngeal elevation. A chin-down posture to push the tongue base posteriorly did not reduce the aspiration.

Suggest continued practice of the supersupraglottic swallow to improve closure of the airway entrance and continued nonoral feeding because of excessive aspiration.

Second outpatient follow-up.   [Name], a 60-year-old man, of [address], was seen for videofluoroscopic reexamination of swallowing on May 28, 1992. [Name] underwent an extended supraglottic laryngectomy 10 weeks ago and has been practicing the supersupraglottic swallow.

During all swallows, [Name] did not use the supersupraglottic swallow. During swallows of 1-ml to 10-ml boluses of thin liquid, paste, and masticated materials, oral transit times were normal with no motility problems. The pharyngeal swallow was triggered normally. No aspiration was seen during the pharyngeal stage of the swallow. Closure of the airway entrance has now improved sufficiently to protect the airway adequately by retraction of the tongue base to contact the anteriorly tilting arytenoid cartilage. Residue remaining in the pharynx after the swallow is now minimal (5% of the bolus). This pattern of functional swallowing was observed on all swallows of all volumes and all consistencies. Suggest full oral intake and discontinuation of the nasogastric tube.

Outpatient Evaluation with One Follow-Up Examination: Closed Head Injury

First outpatient evaluation. [Name], a 24-year-old man, of [address], was seen for a videofluoroscopic examination of oropharyngeal swallow on May 20, 1992. [Name] sustained a closed head injury 3 months ago. In acute care, this patient received a tracheostomy that remained in place for 2 1/2 months. Nutrition is provided through a nasogastric tube.

During swallows of 1 and 3 ml of thin liquid, oral transit times were normal with no motility problems. The pharyngeal swallow was triggered 2 sec late. During the delay, the bolus remained in the valleculae. When the pharyngeal swallow was triggered, laryngeal elevation was reduced, causing residue to remain in the pyriform sinuses. On 3-ml boluses, there was aspiration of the liquid from the pyriform sinuses after the swallow.

[Name] was then laid on his left side to see if changing the direction of gravity would eliminate this aspiration after the swallow. Side-lying with a pillow under the head so that the cervical and thoracic spine were in alignment eliminated the aspiration. On 3-ml to 10-ml boluses and cup drinking of thin liquids, paste, and masticated foods, the residue stayed in the pyriform sinuses, and each succeeding swallow pushed the previous residue into the esophagus so that there was no buildup of material. Repeated swallows of various consistencies were completed in this position with the same results. It is recommended that [name] now initiate oral feeding in the side-lying position and be reevaluated in 1 month in order to assess recovery of pharyngeal contraction.

First outpatient follow-up. [Name], a 24-year-old man, of [address], was seen for videofluoroscopic reexamination of oropharyngeal swallowing on July 15, 1992. [Name] suffered a closed head injury 21 weeks ago and has been eating all meals in a sidelying position for the past 7 weeks. His nasogastric tube was pulled six weeks ago. He reports an 11-pound weight gain and no problems since beginning oral feeding.

During all swallows in the upright position, oral transit times were normal with no motility problems. The pharyngeal swallow was triggered well. During the pharyngeal stage of the swallow, laryngeal elevation was improved and no aspiration was seen. There was minimal residue in the pharynx after the swallow.

[Name] was advised to begin eating in an upright position. He appears to need no more follow-up unless any further problems develop. He has recovered functional swallowing.

Outpatient Evaluation: Total Laryngectomy

[Name], a 58-year-old woman, of [address], was seen for videofluoroscopic examination of oropharyngeal swallowing and esophageal voice production on October 3, 1991. [Name] reported difficulty in learning to put air into the esophagus and release it for esophageal voice, but no swallowing problem.

During swallows of liquid, paste, and masticated material (cookie), oral transit times were normal with no motility problems. Pharyngoesophageal transit appeared to be normal. There was no obstruction in the pharyngoesophagus. There was, however, a very mild pseudoepiglottis at the base of the tongue, which did not appear to narrow the oral pharynx or to restrict passage of a liquid or paste bolus. Thus, swallowing was normal for total laryngectomy.

During attempts to put air into the esophagus for esophageal voice, no air was seen to enter below the adiposed tissue at C4 to C6, the pseudoglottis. The pseudoglottis was located at approximately C4 to C5 and covered a relatively large area. On attempts to improve air intake, such as clucking the tongue or repeated injection, only small amounts of air entered the esophagus and none could be released.

After these attempts by [name] to voluntarily put air into the esophagus, a no. 16 French catheter was inserted through the nose and dropped into the pharyngoesophagus approximately 2 cm below the pseudoglottis. When air was blown through this catheter, a spasm was noted in the pseudoglottis such that air could not be released despite greatly increased air pressure. When the catheter was pulled slightly upward so that the lower end was in the middle of the pseudoglottis, some soft voice was produced. Above the level of the pseudoglottis, only a whisper was elicited.

It appears that [name's] pseudoglottis goes into spasm when air pressure builds up beneath it. Thus, it is physiologically difficult for her to inject and release air and produce any esophageal voice. It is also difficult for her to push air through the segment into the esophagus. At this point it may be worthwhile to consider a myotomy of the pharyngoesophagus to eliminate the spasm in the segment (pseudoglottis) and then to consider tracheoesophageal puncture.

Outpatient Evaluation: Palate-Reshaping Prosthesis

[Name], a 25-year-old woman, of [address], was seen for videofluoroscopic examination of oropharyngeal swallowing on March 8, 1992. She has a mild congenital motor speech disorder with reduced tongue-to-palate contacts during speech. [Name] was seen in the Cleft Palate Clinic and a palate-reshaping prosthesis was recommended for her (Wheeler, Logemann, & Rosen, 1980).

During swallows of liquid, paste, and masticated material (cookie), lingual elevation and contact to the hard palate were reduced. Posterior propulsion of the bolus was slowed. Fine tongue coordination to control the bolus was reduced. The pharyngeal swallow was triggered slightly late. Pharyngeal contraction was reduced, resulting in residue throughout the pharynx (valleculae, pharyngeal walls, and pyriform sinuses) after the swallow. No aspiration was seen.

It appears that a palate-reshaping prosthesis would improve [name's] swallowing by improving tongue-to-palate contacts and speeding oral transit times. The prosthesis should also improve tongue-to-palate contacts for speech.

_N O T E S_

Purchasing Sources for Equipment for Positioning Patients During the Radiographic Procedure

Amigo Escort Video Swallow Chair:
Durable Medical Equipment Shoppe
1600 Shore Road, Unit H
Naperville, IL 60540
(312) 420-7621 or (800) 225-3900

MAMA systems multiple applications and articulations (infant/child chair):
MAMA Systems, Inc.
4347 Silver Lake Street
Oconomowoc, WI 53066
(414) 569-9188

Plywood Sacred Heart Chair (plans):
Manager, Radiation Department
Sacred Heart Hospital
1545 South Layton Boulevard
Milwaukee, WI 53215
(414) 383-4490

Tumble Form Feeder Seats, small, medium, large (Floor Sitter Wedge):
Distributed by J. A. Preston
P.O. Box 89
Jackson, MI 49204
(800) 631-7277

Vess Chair:
Vess Chair, Inc.
2938 North 61st Street
Milwaukee, WI 53210
(414) 932-2203

Video Fluoro Chair:
RehabTech, Inc.
6469 Germantown Pike
Dayton, OH 45418
(513) 866-4308

Video-Fluoroscopic Imaging Chair (VIC):
Hausted, Inc.
927 Lake Road, P.O. Box 710
Medina, OH 44258-0710
(216) 723-3271; FAX: 725-0505

Dsyphagia Journal
Attention: D. Emin
Springer-Verlag New York, Inc.
175 Fifth Avenue
New York, NY 10010

N O T E S

Videofluorographic Worksheet

The purpose of this worksheet is to structure observations of anatomy and physiology made during modified barium swallow (MBS) videofluorographic studies. The worksheet includes the most commonly seen anatomic and physiologic swallowing disorders and leaves space for the examiner to note other disorders seen during the radiographic study. The worksheet focuses on the oral, pharyngeal, and cervical esophageal examination using the MBS procedure (Logemann, 1983). This worksheet has been updated from the one published in *Evaluation and Treatment of Swallowing Disorders* (Logemann, 1983) and the first edition of this manual so that it is easier to use and includes space for documenting data from posterior-anterior (P-A) views as well as lateral views.

The identifying information at the top of the worksheet is designed to provide sufficient room for the clinician to note not only the patient's name and age, but also the date of the radiographic study, the date when oral feeding was initiated in part or totally, the apparent etiology of the patient's swallowing disorder (i.e., the underlying condition causing the swallowing problem, such as stroke or head trauma), the patient's current method of nutritional intake (e.g., oral feeding, nasogastric tube, gastrostomy or jejunostomy), the presence of a tracheostomy tube and the type (e.g., unplugged or cuffed), and the purpose of the radiographic study. The radiographic study may be done to examine the physiology of the swallowing mechanism or to evaluate the effectiveness of a particular treatment strategy or the effects of recovery, and to identify the presence and cause of aspiration.

The worksheet is divided into two sections. The first section is designed for use during swallows of various volumes of liquid. The second section provides room to define swallowing disorders on paste, cookie, and any other foods presented. Each of these two sections is divided into swallow symptoms and disorders viewed videofluorographically in the lateral plane and disorders visible videofluorographically in the P-A plane. In each section, radiographic symptoms are listed in the left column from anterior to posterior and superior to inferior.

Blanks are provided adjacent to each symptom so that the clinician can check the symptoms that are observed during each swallow of a particular volume or consistency. Space is provided to record data from three swallows of five liquid volumes and other consistencies. Although liquid barium (as close to water as possible), pudding containing paste barium (Esophatrast), and cookie coated with barium pudding (representing masticated material) are usually used, the clinician may fill in the name of any consistencies introduced. Clinicians may substitute other food consistencies or omit some consistencies from the evaluation, particularly if a patient is aspirating significantly, despite the introduction of treatment strategies.

Those symptoms that may result in aspiration before, during, or after the swallow are so indicated. Space is provided below each symptom on the sheet for clinical judgment of the amount of aspiration on each swallow.

At the end of each section of the sheet, space is provided to note whether or not any postural intervention or treatment strategy was introduced and its effects on swallowing physiology for various bolus types.

Physiologic disturbances in swallowing that correspond to radiographic symptoms are listed in the far right column, for consideration by the clinician in diagnosing the patient's swallowing disorder.

In the section of the form devoted to notation of observations in the P-A view, space has also been provided for swallows of all bolus types. In fact, often only one or two swallows will be repeated in this P-A view to identify structural or physiologic asymmetries and at the same time minimize the risk of aspiration.

Readers are permitted to reproduce the Videofluorographic Worksheets on the following pages for clinical work and training. Reproduction in any form of any part of the Videofluorographic Worksheets for purposes other than clinical work and training is prohibited.

Videofluorographic Examination of Swallowing
Jeri A. Logemann, PhD, Northwestern University

Patient's name _____ Age _____ Date of study _____ Date oral feeding began _____

Etiology of patient's swallowing disorder _____

Status of nutritional intake _____ Tracheostomy tube _____

Purpose of study _____

Radiographic Symptoms: Lat. View

	Liquids					Possible Swallowing Disorders
Preparation to Swallow	1 ml	3 ml	5 ml	10 ml	Cup	
Cannot hold food in mouth anteriorly	❑❑❑	❑❑❑	❑❑❑	❑❑❑	❑❑❑	Reduced lip closure
Cannot form bolus	❑❑❑	❑❑❑	❑❑❑	❑❑❑	❑❑❑	Red. tongue movement range or coordination
Cannot hold bolus—premature bolus loss	❑❑❑	❑❑❑	❑❑❑	❑❑❑	❑❑❑	Red. tongue shaping/coord.; reduced velar movement
Aspiration (%) before swallow	_____	_____	_____	_____	_____	
Material falls into anterior sulcus	❑❑❑	❑❑❑	❑❑❑	❑❑❑	❑❑❑	Reduced labial tension or tone
Material falls into lateral sulcus	❑❑❑	❑❑❑	❑❑❑	❑❑❑	❑❑❑	Reduced buccal tension or tone
Abnormal hold position	❑❑❑	❑❑❑	❑❑❑	❑❑❑	❑❑❑	Tongue thrust; reduced tongue control
Other_____	❑❑❑	❑❑❑	❑❑❑	❑❑❑	❑❑❑	Describe _____
Posture or treatment introduced	❑❑❑	❑❑❑	❑❑❑	❑❑❑	❑❑❑	Which one? _____
Oral Phase						
Delayed oral onset of swallow	❑❑❑	❑❑❑	❑❑❑	❑❑❑	❑❑❑	Apraxia of swallow; reduced oral sensation
Searching tongue movements	❑❑❑	❑❑❑	❑❑❑	❑❑❑	❑❑❑	Apraxia of swallow
Tongue moves forward to start swallow	❑❑❑	❑❑❑	❑❑❑	❑❑❑	❑❑❑	Tongue thrust
Residue (stasis) in anterior sulcus	❑❑❑	❑❑❑	❑❑❑	❑❑❑	❑❑❑	Reduced labial tension or tone; reduced lingual control
Residue (stasis) in lateral sulcus	❑❑❑	❑❑❑	❑❑❑	❑❑❑	❑❑❑	Reduced buccal tension or tone
Residue (stasis) on floor of mouth	❑❑❑	❑❑❑	❑❑❑	❑❑❑	❑❑❑	Reduced tongue shaping or coordination
Residue in midtongue depression	❑❑❑	❑❑❑	❑❑❑	❑❑❑	❑❑❑	Tongue scarring
Residue (stasis) on tongue	❑❑❑	❑❑❑	❑❑❑	❑❑❑	❑❑❑	Reduced tongue movement; reduced tongue strength
Disturbed lingual contraction	❑❑❑	❑❑❑	❑❑❑	❑❑❑	❑❑❑	Disorganized A-P tongue movement
Incomplete tongue-to-palate contact	❑❑❑	❑❑❑	❑❑❑	❑❑❑	❑❑❑	Reduced tongue elevation
Residue on hard palate	❑❑❑	❑❑❑	❑❑❑	❑❑❑	❑❑❑	Reduced tongue elevation; reduced tongue strength
Reduced A-P tongue movement	❑❑❑	❑❑❑	❑❑❑	❑❑❑	❑❑❑	Reduced A-P lingual coordination
Repetitive lingual rolling actions	❑❑❑	❑❑❑	❑❑❑	❑❑❑	❑❑❑	Parkinson's disease
Uncontrolled bolus/premature swallow	❑❑❑	❑❑❑	❑❑❑	❑❑❑	❑❑❑	Reduced tongue control; reduced linguavelar seal
Aspiration (%) before swallow	_____	_____	_____	_____	_____	(Any reduced tongue control may cause aspiration before swallow)
Piecemeal deglutition	❑❑❑	❑❑❑	❑❑❑	❑❑❑	❑❑❑	May indicate fear of swallowing
Oral transit time (in seconds)	_____	_____	_____	_____	_____	
Other_____	_____	_____	_____	_____	_____	Describe _____
Posture or treatment introduced	❑❑❑	❑❑❑	❑❑❑	❑❑❑	❑❑❑	Which one? _____
Triggering the Pharyngeal Swallow						
Duration of delay (in seconds)	_____	_____	_____	_____	_____	Delayed pharyngeal swallow
% aspiration before swallow	_____	_____	_____	_____	_____	

Radiographic Symptoms   Liquids   Possible Swallowing Disorders

Pharyngeal Phase

Symptom	1 ml	3 ml	5 ml	10 ml	Cup	Possible Swallowing Disorders
Nasal penetration	☐☐☐	☐☐☐	☐☐☐	☐☐☐	☐☐☐	Reduced velopharyngeal closure
Pseudoepiglottis (total laryngect.)	☐☐☐	☐☐☐	☐☐☐	☐☐☐	☐☐☐	Fold of mucosa at base of tongue
Bony outgrowth from cerv. vertebrae	☐☐☐	☐☐☐	☐☐☐	☐☐☐	☐☐☐	Cervical osteophytes
Coating of pharyng. walls after swallow	☐☐☐	☐☐☐	☐☐☐	☐☐☐	☐☐☐	Reduced pharyngeal contraction bilaterally
Vallecular residue (%) after swallow	____	____	____	____	____	Reduced tongue-base posterior movement
Aspiration (%) after swallow	____	____	____	____	____	
Coating in depression on pharyn. wall	☐☐☐	☐☐☐	☐☐☐	☐☐☐	☐☐☐	Scar tissue on pharyngeal wall; pharyn. pouch
Aspiration (%) after swallow	____	____	____	____	____	
Residue at top of airway	☐☐☐	☐☐☐	☐☐☐	☐☐☐	☐☐☐	Reduced laryngeal elevation
Aspiration (%) after swallow	____	____	____	____	____	
Penetration into airway entrance	☐☐☐	☐☐☐	☐☐☐	☐☐☐	☐☐☐	Reduced closure of airway entrance
Aspiration (%) after swallow	____	____	____	____	____	
Aspiration (%) during swallow	____	____	____	____	____	Reduced laryngeal closure
Residue (stasis) in both pyriform sinuses	☐☐☐	☐☐☐	☐☐☐	☐☐☐	☐☐☐	Red. ant. laryngeal motion; cricopharyn. dysfunction; stricture
Aspiration (%) after swallow	____	____	____	____	____	
Residue throughout pharynx	☐☐☐	☐☐☐	☐☐☐	☐☐☐	☐☐☐	Generalized reduction in pressure
Aspiration (%) after swallow	____	____	____	____	____	
Pharyngeal transit time (in seconds)	____	____	____	____	____	
Other_____	☐☐☐	☐☐☐	☐☐☐	☐☐☐	☐☐☐	Describe _____
Posture or treatment introduced	☐☐☐	☐☐☐	☐☐☐	☐☐☐	☐☐☐	Which one? _____

Cervical Esophageal Stage

Symptom	1 ml	3 ml	5 ml	10 ml	Cup	Possible Swallowing Disorders
Esophageal to pharyngeal backflow	☐☐☐	☐☐☐	☐☐☐	☐☐☐	☐☐☐	Esophageal abnormality—further assessment needed
Tracheoesophageal fistula	☐☐☐	☐☐☐	☐☐☐	☐☐☐	☐☐☐	Tracheoesophageal fistula
Zenker's diverticulum	☐☐☐	☐☐☐	☐☐☐	☐☐☐	☐☐☐	Zenker's diverticulum
Other_____	☐☐☐	☐☐☐	☐☐☐	☐☐☐	☐☐☐	Describe _____

P-A View: Preparation to Swallow

Symptom	1 ml	3 ml	5 ml	10 ml	Cup	Possible Swallowing Disorders
Unable to align teeth	☐☐☐	☐☐☐	☐☐☐	☐☐☐	☐☐☐	Reduced mandibular movement
Unable to lateralize material	☐☐☐	☐☐☐	☐☐☐	☐☐☐	☐☐☐	Reduced tongue lateralization
Unable to mash material	☐☐☐	☐☐☐	☐☐☐	☐☐☐	☐☐☐	Reduced tongue elevation
Material falls into lateral sulcus	☐☐☐	☐☐☐	☐☐☐	☐☐☐	☐☐☐	Reduced buccal tension or tone
Material falls to floor of mouth	☐☐☐	☐☐☐	☐☐☐	☐☐☐	☐☐☐	Reduced tongue control
Bolus spread across mouth	☐☐☐	☐☐☐	☐☐☐	☐☐☐	☐☐☐	Reduced fine tongue control
Posture or treatment introduced	☐☐☐	☐☐☐	☐☐☐	☐☐☐	☐☐☐	Which one?

P-A View: Pharyngeal Phase

Symptom	1 ml	3 ml	5 ml	10 ml	Cup	Possible Swallowing Disorders
Unilateral vallecular residue	☐☐☐	☐☐☐	☐☐☐	☐☐☐	☐☐☐	Unilateral dysfunction of tongue base
Residue in one pyriform sinus	☐☐☐	☐☐☐	☐☐☐	☐☐☐	☐☐☐	Unilateral dysfunction of pharynx
____ right—left ____						
Aspiration (%) after swallow	____	____	____	____	____	
Reduced laryngeal movement medially	☐☐☐	☐☐☐	☐☐☐	☐☐☐	☐☐☐	Reduced vocal fold adduction
____ right—left ____						
Aspiration (%) during swallow	____	____	____	____	____	
Unequal height of vocal folds	☐☐☐	☐☐☐	☐☐☐	☐☐☐	☐☐☐	Unequal height of vocal folds
Aspiration (%) during swallow	____	____	____	____	____	
Other_____	☐☐☐	☐☐☐	☐☐☐	☐☐☐	☐☐☐	Describe _____
Posture or treatment introduced	☐☐☐	☐☐☐	☐☐☐	☐☐☐	☐☐☐	Which one? _____

Radiographic Symptoms

Lateral View	1 ml			Other		Possible Swallowing Disorders
Preparation to Swallow	Paste	Cookie	_____	_____	_____	
Cannot hold food in mouth anteriorly	☐☐☐	☐☐☐	☐☐☐	☐☐☐	☐☐☐	Reduced lip closure
Cannot form bolus	☐☐☐	☐☐☐	☐☐☐	☐☐☐	☐☐☐	Red. tongue movement range or coordination
Cannot hold bolus—premature bolus loss	☐☐☐	☐☐☐	☐☐☐	☐☐☐	☐☐☐	Red. tongue shaping/coord.; reduced palatal movement
Aspiration (%) before swallow	_____	_____	_____	_____	_____	
Material falls into anterior sulcus	☐☐☐	☐☐☐	☐☐☐	☐☐☐	☐☐☐	Reduced labial tension or tone
Material falls into lateral sulcus	☐☐☐	☐☐☐	☐☐☐	☐☐☐	☐☐☐	Reduced buccal tension or tone
Abnormal hold position	☐☐☐	☐☐☐	☐☐☐	☐☐☐	☐☐☐	Tongue thrust; reduced tongue control
Other_____	☐☐☐	☐☐☐	☐☐☐	☐☐☐	☐☐☐	Describe _____
Posture or treatment introduced	☐☐☐	☐☐☐	☐☐☐	☐☐☐	☐☐☐	Which one? _____
Oral Phase						
Delayed oral onset of swallow	☐☐☐	☐☐☐	☐☐☐	☐☐☐	☐☐☐	Apraxia of swallow; reduced oral sensation
Searching tongue movements	☐☐☐	☐☐☐	☐☐☐	☐☐☐	☐☐☐	Apraxia of swallow
Tongue moves forward to start swallow	☐☐☐	☐☐☐	☐☐☐	☐☐☐	☐☐☐	Tongue thrust
Residue (stasis) in anterior sulcus	☐☐☐	☐☐☐	☐☐☐	☐☐☐	☐☐☐	Reduced labial tension or tone; reduced lingual control
Residue (stasis) in lateral sulcus	☐☐☐	☐☐☐	☐☐☐	☐☐☐	☐☐☐	Reduced buccal tension or tone
Residue (stasis) on floor of mouth	☐☐☐	☐☐☐	☐☐☐	☐☐☐	☐☐☐	Reduced tongue shaping or coordination
Residue in midtongue depression	☐☐☐	☐☐☐	☐☐☐	☐☐☐	☐☐☐	Tongue scarring
Residue (stasis) on tongue	☐☐☐	☐☐☐	☐☐☐	☐☐☐	☐☐☐	Reduced tongue movement; reduced tongue strength
Disturbed lingual contraction	☐☐☐	☐☐☐	☐☐☐	☐☐☐	☐☐☐	Disorganized A-P tongue movement
Incomplete tongue-to-palate contact	☐☐☐	☐☐☐	☐☐☐	☐☐☐	☐☐☐	Reduced tongue elevation
Residue on hard palate	☐☐☐	☐☐☐	☐☐☐	☐☐☐	☐☐☐	Reduced tongue elevation; reduced tongue strength
Reduced A-P tongue movement	☐☐☐	☐☐☐	☐☐☐	☐☐☐	☐☐☐	Reduced A-P lingual coordination
Repetitive lingual rolling actions	☐☐☐	☐☐☐	☐☐☐	☐☐☐	☐☐☐	Parkinson's disease
Uncontrolled bolus/premature swallow	☐☐☐	☐☐☐	☐☐☐	☐☐☐	☐☐☐	Reduced tongue control; reduced linguavelar seal
Aspiration (%) before swallow	_____	_____	_____	_____	_____	(Any reduced tongue control may cause aspiration before swallow)
Piecemeal deglutition	☐☐☐	☐☐☐	☐☐☐	☐☐☐	☐☐☐	May indicate fear of swallowing
Oral transit time (in seconds)	_____	_____	_____	_____	_____	
Other_____	_____	_____	_____	_____	_____	Describe _____
Posture or treatment introduced	☐☐☐	☐☐☐	☐☐☐	☐☐☐	☐☐☐	Which one? _____
Triggering the Pharyngeal swallow						
Duration of delay (in seconds)	_____	_____	_____	_____	_____	Delayed pharyngeal swallow
% aspiration before swallow	_____	_____	_____	_____	_____	

Pharyngeal Phase	1 ml	3 ml	5 ml	10 ml	Cookie	**Possible Swallowing Disorders**
Nasal penetration	☐☐☐	☐☐☐	☐☐☐	☐☐☐	☐☐☐	Reduced velopharyngeal closure
Pseudoepiglottis (total laryngect.)	☐☐☐	☐☐☐	☐☐☐	☐☐☐	☐☐☐	Fold of mucosa at base of tongue
Bony outgrowth from cerv. vertebrae	☐☐☐	☐☐☐	☐☐☐	☐☐☐	☐☐☐	Cervical osteophytes

Radiographic Symptoms

	1 ml			Other		Possible Swallowing Disorders
Pharyngeal Phase (continued)	Paste	Cookie	_____	_____	_____	
Coating of pharyng. walls after swallow	□□□	□□□	□□□	□□□	□□□	Reduced pharyngeal contraction bilaterally
Vallecular residue (%) after swallow	_____	_____	_____	_____	_____	Reduced tongue-base posterior movement
Aspiration (%) after swallow	_____	_____	_____	_____	_____	
Coating in depression on pharyn. wall	□□□	□□□	□□□	□□□	□□□	Scar tissue on pharyngeal wall; pharyn. pouch
Aspiration (%) after swallow	_____	_____	_____	_____	_____	
Residue at top of airway	□□□	□□□	□□□	□□□	□□□	Reduced laryngeal elevation
Aspiration (%) after swallow	_____	_____	_____	_____	_____	
Penetration into airway entrance	□□□	□□□	□□□	□□□	□□□	Reduced closure of airway entrance
Aspiration (%) after swallow	_____	_____	_____	_____	_____	
Aspiration (%) during swallow	_____	_____	_____	_____	_____	Reduced laryngeal closure
Residue (stasis) in both pyriform sinuses	□□□	□□□	□□□	□□□	□□□	Red. ant. laryngeal motion; cricopharyn. dysfunction; stricture
Aspiration (%) after swallow	_____	_____	_____	_____	_____	
Residue throughout pharynx	□□□	□□□	□□□	□□□	□□□	Generalized reduction in pressure
Aspiration (%) after swallow	_____	_____	_____	_____	_____	
Pharyngeal transit time (in seconds)	_____	_____	_____	_____		
Other_____	□□□	□□□	□□□	□□□	□□□	Describe _____
Posture or treatment introduced	□□□	□□□	□□□	□□□	□□□	Which one? _____

Cervical Esophageal Stage

Esophageal to pharyngeal backflow	□□□	□□□	□□□	□□□	□□□	Esophageal abnormality—further assessment needed
Tracheoesophageal fistula	□□□	□□□	□□□	□□□	□□□	Tracheoesophageal fistula
Zenker's diverticulum	□□□	□□□	□□□	□□□	□□□	Zenker's diverticulum
Other_____	□□□	□□□	□□□	□□□	□□□	Describe _____

P-A View: Preparation to Swallow

Unable to align teeth	□□□	□□□	□□□	□□□	□□□	Reduced mandibular movement
Unable to lateralize material	□□□	□□□	□□□	□□□	□□□	Reduced tongue lateralization
Unable to mash material	□□□	□□□	□□□	□□□	□□□	Reduced tongue elevation
Material falls into lateral sulcus	□□□	□□□	□□□	□□□	□□□	Reduced buccal tension or tone
Material falls to floor of mouth	□□□	□□□	□□□	□□□	□□□	Reduced tongue control
Bolus spread across mouth	□□□	□□□	□□□	□□□	□□□	Reduced fine tongue control
Posture or treatment introduced	□□□	□□□	□□□	□□□	□□□	Which one? _____

P-A View: Pharyngeal Phase

Unilateral vallecular residue	□□□	□□□	□□□	□□□	□□□	Unilateral dysfunction of tongue base
Residue in one pyriform sinus	□□□	□□□	□□□	□□□	□□□	Unilateral dysfunction of pharynx
_____ right—left _____						
Aspiration (%) after swallow	_____	_____	_____	_____	_____	
Reduced laryngeal movement medially	□□□	□□□	□□□	□□□	□□□	Reduced vocal fold adduction
_____ right—left _____						
Aspiration (%) during swallow	_____	_____	_____	_____	_____	
Unequal height of vocal folds	□□□	□□□	□□□	□□□	□□□	Unequal height of vocal folds
Aspiration (%) during swallow	_____	_____	_____	_____	_____	
Other_____	□□□	□□□	□□□	□□□	□□□	Describe _____
Posture or treatment introduced	□□□	□□□	□□□	□□□	□□□	Which one? _____

Audiovisual Aids Available on Swallowing and Swallowing Disorders

Title: *Acquired Dysphagias: Case Studies with Videofluoroscopic Analysis*

Prepared by: Linda Susan Day, MA, CCC-SP, and Mary Tougher, MS, CCC-SP

Available from: University of Missouri–Columbia, Speech and Hearing Clinic
                  125 Parker Hall, Columbia, MO 65211

Options: Rent (10 days) ½″ or ¾″ Beta or VHS videotape or purchase ½″ or
                  ¾″ videotape

Description: Presents a variety of acquired dysphagic conditions (13 case stud-
                  ies). Cases demonstrate typical patterns of dysphagic symptoms in
                  most common neuropathologies as well as those found in less com-
                  monly encountered conditions. Includes evaluation, videofluoro-
                  scopic examination, treatment plan, and case outcome.

Title: *The Normal Pharyngeal Swallow*

Prepared by: Martin Donner, Chair, Radiology Department, Johns Hopkins
                  Hospital

Available from: Johns Hopkins Hospital, Baltimore, MD 21205, (301) 955-3562

Options: Purchase 16mm film; rent (1 week) or purchase videotape

Description: The anatomy, physiology, and neuroregulation of the normal degluti-
                  tion sequence demonstrated by cinefluorography and animation.

Title: *Videofluoroscopic Assessment of Dysphagia in Neuromotor Disorders*

Prepared by: Shaun Brayton-Gerratt, MA, CCC, and Bruce Gerratt, PhD

Produced by: Carondelet Rehabilitation Centers of America

Available from: Medical Electronic Educational Services, Inc.,
                  P.O. Box 50700, Tucson, AZ 85703, (602) 624-4401

Description: Videotape contains segments of radiographic studies of normal
                  patients and individuals with variety of physiologic abnormalities.
                  Narrated by a radiologist and a speech language pathologist.

Title: *Videofluoroscopic Evaluation of Swallowing Dysfunction*

Prepared by: Lisa Newman, MA, CCC-SP, Thomas Anderson, MD, and Philip Caligiuri, MD

Available from: Mercy Hospital and Medical Center, Speech Language Pathology Department
                  2510 South King Drive, Chicago, IL 60616, (312) 567-5650

Options: Rent (2 weeks) or purchase VHS ½″ or U-Matic ¾″ videocassette

Description: Exemplifies technical aspects of fluoroscopic procedures for swallowing studies, reviews normal swallowing process, and includes three sample evaluations. Suitable for speech language pathologists, radiologists, and other medical personnel concerned with swallowing disorders.

Titles prepared by: Jeri A. Logemann, PhD, Northwestern University, Evanston, IL 60208

Available from: Northern Speech Services, Inc.
                     304 Grandview Boulevard, P.O. Box 544, Gaylord, MI 49735, (517) 732-3866

Assessment of Swallowing Physiology: Videofluorographic Study of Oropharyngeal Deglutition

Options: Manual + 40 slides + 55-minute ¾″ videotape
               Manual + 40 slides + 55-minute ½″ videotape
               Manual + 55-minute ¾″ videotape
               Manual + 55-minute ½″ videotape
               Manual + 40 slides

Description: This 55-minute videotape and/or 40-slide program presents the technique for videofluorographic examination of oropharyngeal deglutition including equipment, implements, supplies, patient positioning, procedure for examination, and application of compensatory strategies and therapy techniques.

The Management of Swallowing Disorders: An Inservice Training Program

Options: 20-minute ¾″ videotape or 20-minute ½″ videotape
               Manual + 30 slides
               Manual + 30 slides + ½″ videotape
               Manual + 30 slides + ¾″ videotape

Description: Twenty-minute videotape; 30 slides and videotape presentation designed for lectures and inservice education with physicians, nurses, and other health care professionals. Contains illustrations and information on the anatomy and physiology of normal swallowing, the radiographic procedure known as the modified barium swallow, and management and treatment techniques such as posture and thermal stimulation. Answers such frequently asked questions as "Can the gag reflex predict the swallow?" "What is the difference between the barium swallow and the modified barium swallow?" and "What can the modified barium swallow tell us that we can't see in the barium swallow?"

Physiologic and Anatomic Oropharyngeal Swallowing Disorders

Options: 55-minute ¾″ videotape + manual
55-minute ½″ videotape + manual

Description: Contains real-time and slow-motion narrated examples of normal swallowing and oral and pharyngeal disorders, as well as 15 unnarrated test samples. The manual describes the various disorders, provides sample reports for the 15 test items, and includes a section on radiographic anatomy including a self-test.

Precautions for Feeding Dysphagic Patients: An Inservice Training Program for Feeding Staff

Options: 25-minute ½″ videotape + 50 manuals and Feeding Plan forms (ship. about $14)
25-minute ¾″ videotape + 50 manuals and Feeding Plan forms (ship. about $14)

Description: This 25-minute videotape, manual, and Individualized Feeding Plan form describe the aspects of feeding that should be monitored to assure the safest oral intake for patients with swallowing problems and gives the rationale for particular feeding procedures; tape and manual briefly describe and illustrate normal swallowing physiology.

_N O T E S_

References

Aronson, A. (1981). Early motor unit disease masquerading as psychogenic breathy dysphonia: A clinical case presentation. *Journal of Speech and Hearing Disorders, 36,* 116–124.

Bisch, E., Logemann, J., Rademaker, A., & Quigley, J. (1992). *Swallow effects of the SOMI brace.* Paper presented at the American Speech-Language-Hearing Association annual convention, San Antonio, TX.

Blonsky, R., Logemann, J., Boshes, B., & Fisher, H. (1978). Comparison of speech and swallowing function in patients with tremor disorders and in normal geriatric patients: A cinefluorographic study. *Journal of Gerontology, 30,* 299–303.

Bosma, J. F. (1986). Development of feeding. *Clinical Nutrition, 5,* 210–218.

Cerenko, D., McConnel, F. M. S., & Jackson, R. T. (1989). Quantitative assessment of pharyngeal bolus driving forces. *Otolaryngology—Head & Neck Surgery, 100,* 57–63.

Cook, I. J., Dodds, W. J., Dantas, R. O., Kern, M. K., Massey, B. T., Shaker, R., & Hogan, W. J. (1989). Timing of videofluoroscopic, manometric events, and bolus transit during the oral and pharyngeal phases of swallowing. *Dysphagia, 4,* 8–15.

Cook, I. J., Dodds, W. J., Dantas, R. O., Massey, B., Kern, M. K., Lang, I. M., Brasseur, I. G., & Hogan, W. J. (1989). Opening mechanisms of the human upper esophageal sphincter. *American Journal of Physiology, 257 (Gastrointestinal and Liver Physiology 20),* G748–G759.

Dantas, R. O., Dodds, W. J., Massey, B. T., & Kern, M. K. (1989). The effect of high vs. low density barium preparations on the quantitative features of swallowing. *American Journal of Radiology, 153,* 1191–1195.

Dantas, R. O., Kern, M. K., Massey, B. T., Dodds, W. J., Kahrilas, P. J., Brasseur, J. G., Cook, I. J., & Lang, I. M. (1990). Effect of swallowed bolus variables on oral and pharyngeal phases of swallowing. *American Journal of Physiology, 258 (Gastrointestinal and Liver Physiology),* G675–G681.

Dodds, W. J., Hogan, W. J., Lydon, S. B., Stewart, E. T., Stef, J. J., & Arndorfer, R. C. (1975). Quantification of pharyngeal motor function in normal human subjects. *Journal of Applied Physiology, 39,* 692–696.

Dodds, W., Hogan, W., Reid, D., Stewart, E., & Arndorfer, R. (1973). A comparison between primary esophageal peristalsis following wet and dry swallows. *Journal of Applied Physiology, 35(6),* 850–857.

Dodds, W. J., Logemann, J. A., & Stewart, E. T. (1990). Radiological assessment of abnormal oral and pharyngeal phases of swallowing. *American Journal of Roentgenology, 154,* 965–974.

Dodds, W. J., Man, K. M., Cook, I. J., Kahrilas, P. J., Stewart, E. T., & Kern, M. K. (1988). Influence of bolus volume on swallow-induced hyoid movement in normal subjects. *American Journal of Roentgenology, 150,* 1307–1309.

Dodds, W. J., Stewart, E. T., & Logemann, J. (1990). Physiology and radiology of the normal oral and pharyngeal phases of swallowing. *American Journal of Roentgenology, 154,* 953–963.

Dodds, W. J., Taylor, A. J., Stewart, E. T., Kern, M. K., Logemann, J. A., & Cook, I. J. (1989). Tipper and dipper types of oral swallows. *American Journal of Roentgenology, 153,* 1197–1199.

Donner, M. W., & Silbiger, M. L. (1966). Cinefluorographic analysis of swallowing in neuromuscular disorders. *Journal of American Medical Science, 251,* 600–616.

Doty, R. W. (1968). Neural organization of deglutition. In C. F. Code (Ed.), *Handbook of physiology, alimentary canal* (Sec. 5, Vol. 4, pp.1861–1902). Washington, DC: American Physiological Society.

Horner, J., Massey, E. W., Riski, J. E., Lathrop, D., & Chase, K. N. (1988). Aspiration following stroke: Clinical correlates and outcomes. *Neurology, 38,* 1359–1362.

Jacob, P., Kahrilas, P. J., Logemann, J. A., Shah, V., & Ha, T. (1989). Upper esophageal sphincter opening and modulation during swallowing. *Gastroenterology, 97,* 1469–1478.

Kahrilas, P. J., Dodds, W. J., Dent, J., Logemann, J. A., & Shaker, R. (1988). Upper esophageal sphincter function during deglutition. *Gastroenterology, 95,* 52–62.

Kahrilas, P. J., Lin, S., Logemann, J. A., Ergun, G. A., & Facchini, F. 1993. Deglutitive tongue action: Volume accommodation and bolus propulsion. *Gastroenterology, 104,* 152–162.

Kahrilas, P. J., Logemann, J. A., Krugler, C., & Flanagan, E. (1991). Volitional augmentation of upper esophageal sphincter opening during swallowing. *American Journal of Physiology, 260 (Gastrointestinal and Liver Physiology, 23),* G450–G456.

Kahrilas, P. J., Logemann, J. A., Lin, S., & Ergun, G. A. (1992). Pharyngeal clearance during swallowing: A combined manometric and videofluoroscopic study. *Gastroenterology, 103,* 128–136.

Kirchner, J. A. (1967). Pharyngeal and esophageal dysfunction: The diagnosis. *Minnesota Medicine, 50,* 921–924.

Lazzara, G., Lazarus, C., & Logemann, J. (1986). Impact of thermal stimulation on the triggering of the pharyngeal swallow. *Dysphagia, 1,* 73–77.

Lazarus, C., & Logemann, J. (1987). Swallowing disorders in closed head trauma patients. *Archives of Physical Medicine and Rehabilitation, 68,* 79–87.

Linden P., & Siebens A. (1983). Dysphagia: Predicting laryngeal penetration. *Archives of Physical Medicine and Rehabilitation, 64,* 281–284.

Logemann, J. (1983). *Evaluation and treatment of swallowing disorders.* Austin, TX: PRO-ED.

Logemann, J. (1985). Aspiration in head and neck surgical patients. *Annals of Otology, Rhinology and Laryngology, 94,* 373–376.

Logemann, J. (1986). Treatment for aspiration related to dysphagia: An overview. *Dysphagia, 1,* 34–38.

Logemann, J. (1989a). Deglutition disorders in cancer of the head and neck. In R. Kagan & J. Miles (Eds.), *Head and neck oncology* (pp. 155–161). Philadelphia: B. C. Decker.

Logemann, J. (Ed.). (1989b). Oral intake disorders after head injury. *Journal of Head Trauma Rehabilitation, 4*(4), 24–33.

Logemann, J. A. (1990a). Effects of aging on the swallowing mechanism. In G. Sisson & H. Pelzer (Eds.), *The otolaryngologic clinics of North America: Head and neck diseases in the elderly* (Vol. 23, No. 6, pp. 1045–1056). Philadelphia: W. B. Saunders.

Logemann, J. (1990b). Normal swallowing and the effects of oral cancer on normal deglutition. In W. Fee, H. Geopfert, M. Johns, E. Strong, & P. Ward (Eds.), *Head and neck cancer* (Vol. 2, pp. 324–326). Toronto: B. C. Decker.

Logemann, J. A., & Kahrilas, P. J. (1990). Relearning to swallow after stroke—application of maneuvers and indirect biofeedback: A case study. *Neurology, 40,* 1136–1138.

Logemann, J. A., Kahrilas, P. J., Begelman, J., Dodds, W. J., & Pauloski, B. R. (1989). Interactive computer program for biomechanical analysis of videoradiographic studies of swallowing. *American Journal of Roentgenology, 153,* 277–280.

Logemann, J. A., Kahrilas, P. J., Cheng, J., Pauloski, B. R., Gibbons, P. J., Rademaker, A. W., & Lin, S. (1992). Closure mechanisms of laryngeal vestibule during swallow. *American Journal of Physiology, 262 (Gastrointestinal and Liver Physiology, 25),* G338–G344.

Logemann, J., Kahrilas, P., Kobara, M., & Vakil, N. (1989). The benefit of head rotation on pharyngeal dysphagia. *Archives of Physical Medicine and Rehabilitation, 70,* 767–771.

Mandelstam, P., & Lieber, A. (1970). A cineradiographic evaluation of the esophagus in normal adults. *Gastroenterology, 58,* 32–38.

Martin, B. (1991). *The influence of deglutition on respiration.* Unpublished doctoral dissertation, Northwestern University, Evanston, IL.

McConnel, F. M. S., Hester, R., Mendelsohn, J., & Logemann, J. A. (1988). Manofluorography of deglutition after total laryngopharyngectomy. *Plastic and Reconstructive Surgery, 81*(3), 346–351.

McConnel, F. M. S., Mendelsohn, J., & Logemann, J. (1986). Examination of swallowing after total laryngectomy using manofluorography. *Head & Neck Surgery, 9,* 3–12.

McConnel, F. M. S., Mendelsohn, J., & Logemann, J. (1987). Manofluorography of deglutition after supraglottic laryngectomy. *Head & Neck Surgery, 10,* 142–150.

Miller, A. (1982). Deglutition. *Physiologic Reviews, 62,* 129–184.

Morris, S. E. (1982). *The normal acquisition of oral feeding skills: Implications for assessment and treatment* (pp. 24–32). Central Islip, NY: Therapeutic Media, Inc.

Newman, L. A., Cleveland, R. H., Blickman, J. G., Hillman, R. E., & Jaramillo, D. (1991). Videofluoroscopic analysis of the infant swallow. *Investigative Radiology, 26,* 870–873.

Pommerenke, W. (1928). A study of the sensory areas eliciting the pharyngeal swallow. *American Journal of Physiology, 84,* 36–44.

Rademaker, A. W., Logemann, J. A., Pauloski, B. R., Bowman, J. B., Lazarus, C. L., Sisson, G. A., Milianti, F. J., Graner, D., Cook, B. S., Collins, S. L., Stein, D. W., Beery, Q. C., Johnson, J. T., & Baker, T. M. (1993). Recovery of postoperative swallowing in patients undergoing partial laryngectomy. *Head and Neck* (in press).

Rasley, A., Logemann, J. A., Kahrilas, P. J., Rademaker, A. W., Pauloski, B. R., & Dodds, W. J. (in press). Management of aspiration during the videofluoroscopic study of oropharyngeal dysphagia. *American Journal of Roentgenology.*

Robbins, J. A. (1987). Swallowing in ALS and motor neuron disorders. *Neurologic Clinics, 5,* 213–229.

Robbins, J., & Levine, R. (1988). Swallowing after unilateral stroke of the cerebral cortex: Preliminary experience. *Dysphagia, 3,* 11–17.

Robbins, J. A., Hamilton, J. W., Lof, G. L., & Kempster, G. B. (1992). Oropharyngeal swallowing in normal adults of different ages. *Gastroenterology, 103,* 823–829.

Robbins, J. A., Logemann, J. A., & Kirshner, H. S. (1986). Swallowing and speech production in Parkinson's disease. *Annals of Neurology, 19,* 283–287.

Sessions, D., Zil, R., & Schwartz, S. (1979). Deglutition after conservation surgery for cancer of the larynx and hypopharynx. *Otolaryngology, Head and Neck Surgery, 87,* 779–796.

Shanahan, T. K., Logemann, J. A., Rademaker, A. W., Pauloski, B. R., & Kahrilas, P. J. (in press). Effects of chin-down posture on aspiration in dysphagic patients. *Archives of Physical Medicine and Rehabilitation.*

Shawker, T., Sonies, B., Stone, M., & Baum, G. (1983). Real-time ultrasound visualization of tongue movement during swallowing. *Journal of Clinical Ultrasound, 11,* 485–494.

Shedd, D., Scatliff, J., & Kirchner, J. (1960). The buccopharyngeal propulsive mechanism in human deglutition. *Surgery, 48,* 846–853.

Sonies, B. C., Baum, B. J., & Shawker, T. H. (1984). Tongue motion in elderly adults: Initial in situ observations. *Journal of Gerontology, 39*(3), 279–283.

Sonies, B., Parent, L., Morrish, K., & Baum, B. (1988). Durational aspects of the oral-pharyngeal phase of swallow in normal adults. *Dysphagia, 3,* 1–10.

Tracy, J. F., Logemann, J. A., Kahrilas, P. J., Jacob, P., Kobara, M., & Krugler, C. (1989). Preliminary observations on the effects of age on oropharyngeal deglutition. *Dysphagia, 4,* 90–94.

Tuch, B. E., & Nielsen, J. M. (1941). Apraxia of swallowing. *Bulletin of Los Angeles Neurologic Society, 6,* 52–54.

Veis, S. & Logemann, J. (1985). The nature of swallowing disorders in CVA patients. *Archives of Physical Medicine and Rehabilitation, 66,* 372–375.

Welch, M. W., Logemann, J. A., Rademaker, A. W., & Kahrilas, P. J. (1993). Changes in pharyngeal dimensions effected by chin tuck. *Archives of Physical Medicine and Rehabilitation, 74,* 170–177.

Wheeler, R., Logemann, J., & Rosen, M. (1980). Maxillary reshaping prosthesis: Effectiveness in improving speech and swallowing of post-surgical oral cancer patients. *Journal of Prosthetic Dentistry, 43,* 313–320.

Ylvisaker, M., & Logemann, J. A. (1986). Therapy for feeding and swallowing following head injury. In M. Ylvisaker (Ed.), *Management of head injured patients.* San Diego: College-Hill.